Having a Showdown with Mental Illness

by

Mary Khazak Grant

Dedicated to

LeAnn Nelson, L.C.S.W.

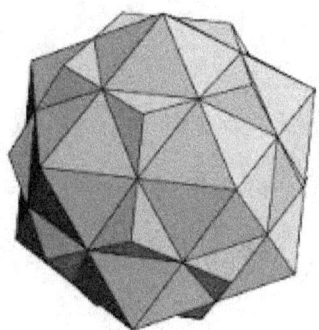

Reality? Hmmmm...

Introduction-

This book is meant as a guide primarily for the individual who has suffered from chronic mental illness. What follows is but a guide for self-help in overcoming mental illness. It offers suggestions, and is not meant to be a guaranteed means to a sure recovery. In the author's case, it apparently worked--what follows is her testimony.

The author developed a method of cure by necessity. It was tested and succeeded in putting her back on her feet. Frustrated by years of conventional therapy, she gained valuable insights while earning a B.A. in Psychology and applied them to her own problems.

This is only offered as a supplement to your own medical regimen. There is no guarantee, of course, that applying suggestions from the author will cure you once and for all of your mental affliction. To help is the intent--she can only attest to an apparent success in her own case. The author is now a fulfilled and productive human being, quite proud of her accomplishments in both the professional and personal arena.

We are all unique. Use this book to develop your own strategy for curing yourself!

About the organization of this book—The first part of the book presents the recommended program to follow. Part Two will have chapters organized by useful topic. It is derived from my *marykhazakgrant.wordpress.com* blog, developed from 2013 to the present. This is organized by topics of pertinent interest to those in recovery. It depicts obstacles crossed in recovery, realistic solutions to problems, and mature perspectives on mental illness which hopefully, you will find very helpful.

PART ONE: THE PROGRAM—WORK COMMENCES

Chapter 1: Patience

Patience is key. You are going in for a consuming battle which will last twenty years or more. No one cares about you as much as you!

At the other side of the wall of stigma, when you've managed to remove those distorted goggles and break them, when fresh cool air is pouring in, "baby" has a new wardrobe, you've connected emotionally with a new man or woman and you're assured, on your feet--is a chance, a second one.

Patience is a virtue. You're the war-torn veteran. Other people won't know where you've been, but you know you were there. The wrinkles on your brow reveal it. So you're now a very good person, but at times feel like a "retread", like someone starting over once more.

So you're a little overly serious, a little more motivated to succeed than most people. That's because you had to over-train good habits, and had to overcompensate for weaknesses. A little discipline wouldn't hurt them either!

Stand tall! You've beat the odds. With chronic mental illness, only one person in twenty ever makes a full recovery or is considered cured. Now, throw your checkbook away, the one you paid therapists with. And throw away your crutches, once and for all.

Don't look in the mirror at the face, with those extra brow lines, the deep circles under the eyes, or the now graying hair. You've lost a lot of time, it's true. Now, you can catch up! Those goals! Dust them off!

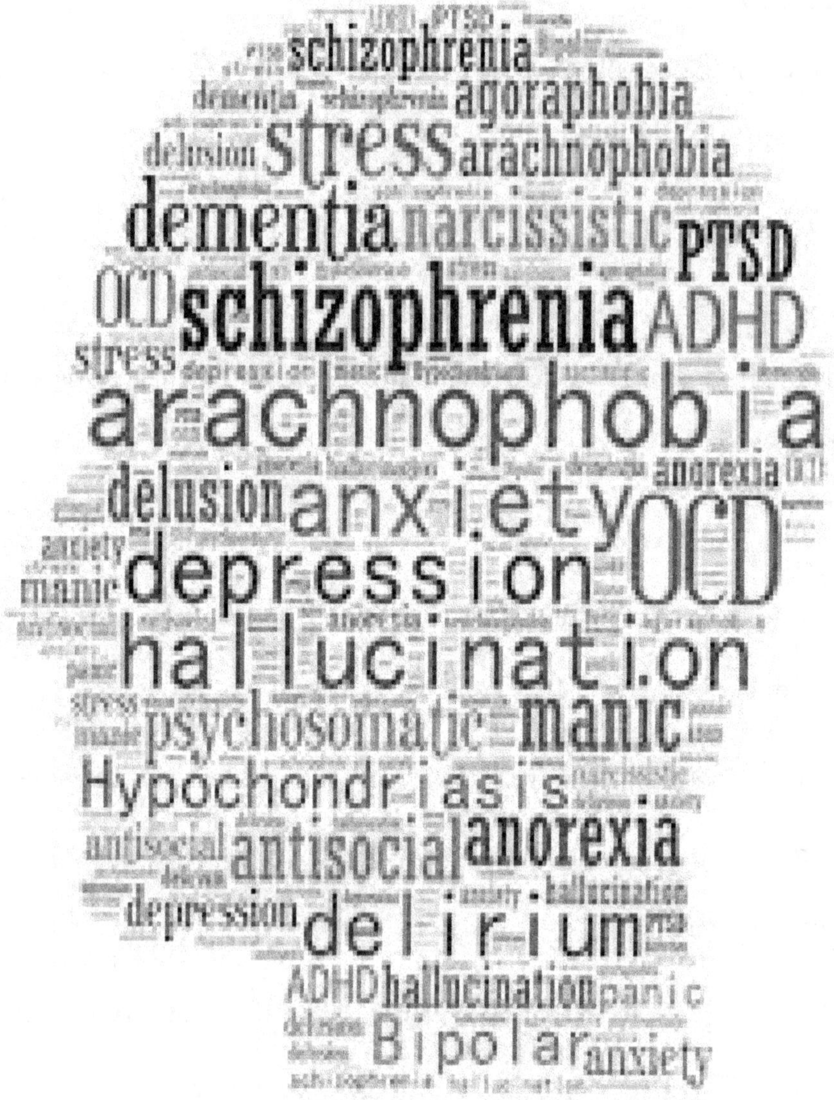
PTSD
schizophrenia
Bipolar
dementia
schizophrenia
agoraphobia
delusion
stress
arachnophobia
dementia
narcissistic
PTSD
OCD
schizophrenia
ADHD
stress
arachnophobia
anorexia
delusion
anxiety
OCD
anxiety
manic
depression
hallucination
stress
manic
psychosomatic
manic
Hypochondriasis
antisocial
antisocial
anorexia
anxiety
hallucination
depression
delirium
ADHD
hallucination
panic
Bipolar
anxiety
schizophrenia

Chapter 2: Where To Start Work

After that long battle which I've mentioned, the patient uphill climb, though bumpy--and you've gotten enough balance chemically and emotionally--you enter a predisposed "cured" phase.   Please note that it might take 17 years to reach this point in your therapy.

The human brain has a resiliency and capacity to recover from those agents, traumas or conditions which, in a predisposed person, led to the disruption we call mental illness. In a sense, that takes up residence in your soul and your perceptual matrix is stretched, distorted or fragmented.

Nothing can't be undone when it concerns a human brain.   I speak from long experience. After years of hallucinations and delusions, my brain shucked off the mentally ill viewpoint.

There, on the "other side", maybe like myself you've cured your chronic, genetic tendency to destabilize.   You threw out the things in the environment which did it to you--and this might be a parent, or a habit to overspend. There are many ways to find a new footing.

And you've been medication-freed, you're on vacation from it--_the sign being a stubborn tendency to push away helpers.   Yet, that bottle of medicine is still in the bathroom cabinet, ready for use should you find the new reality unbearable.   But—you've pushed away your emotional crutches and walked.   That must be supported...and if not, there's another delay in recovery, a serious one.

You've balanced. You're in *New Balance*® shoes, so to speak. Like a mummy, you watch as your doctor approaches you, removing the gauze wrapped around your head--and you've got a new head on.   It really is a break with the past. You feel and act differently.

My friend, your neurotransmitters are now the equal to a racehorse's!   Although it is true that medical science cannot yet adequately explain why certain drugs work—they nevertheless affect your brain chemistry for the good.   There is carryover after the medications are removed.

You've over-learned to be well. Your body has habituated itself to health.   You do everything you can to stabilize—it's a personal and predominant job title.

As a result, you are stronger by far than most people.   You merely need to tap into it.

We are going to now devise a plan together to help you face future challenges, similar to a runner's training program.

See your new self in the mirror!   You are sensitive, with both new skin and new eyes--you don't know your new self, though, fully.

And since you've probably been sex-deprived for years, you might wish to start with your serious remaining flaw: your retarded social skills.

So, let's start the next chapter with that.

Chapter 3: The Attitude

There are people out here who get ahead simply because they destabilize people who compete with them.

They are like bullies kicking sand in all the faces of "90-pound weaklings".

It's foolish to think the world is protective. Face it before you go back out there. It's not going to be as soft as the couch your talk therapist gave you.

People probing your vulnerabilities who may know and even make use of your history are going to, as you begin to progress toward independent rewards, treat you like a marked man or woman. Don't be fooled. They fight dirty. They do destabilize as a tactic. There is a stigma.

You were unaware of this, right?

This is just the first social skill to acquire which all people already have: the art of self-defense.

Sign up for a martial arts program to get a taste of the attitude, all right? Martial arts will toughen up your attitude toward the world. It'll give you a concrete means to protect yourself.

You've made yourself vulnerable to a therapist in order to probe your psyche. For years, it was necessary to work out those conflicts, delusions, and hallucinations. This is not a habit you want to maintain in recovery. Time to close the door! Perhaps you might be soft and open with a loved one in the future. But in all other cases, you need some psychological body armor.

Yes, I'm very serious.   Judo. Karate. Kick-boxing. Wrestling.

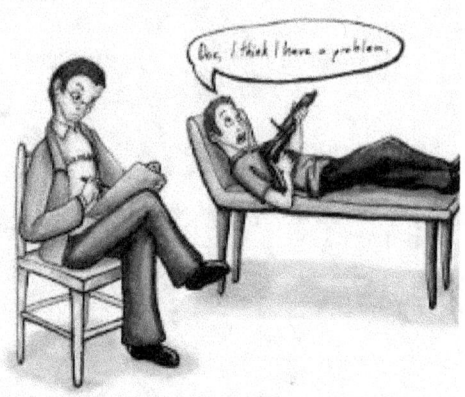

Chapter 4: Confidence Is Key

Being strong is conditional. You will be amazed at how a little something going wrong in the environment will hit you in your *savior faire*.

You must be cautious. Seeking to avoid a false sense of confidence is wise. People will appreciate honesty. Don't be afraid to admit there was a psychological break, you acted out for a day, or that your outburst was possibly due to a previous incident.

But also: do not be trod upon, nor used or worn down. Do not be set back by a moment or two of "flashbacks". And do not be shaken in confidence regarding whether or not you are a well person.

A weak moment, a comment taken the wrong way, is only an opening for someone like a friend, used to passing you your crutch, to return to his well-played role. Don't encourage that. Be realistic, but train him firmly.

You don't need unwanted stress. You must avoid stress situations, but don't compromise your goals and desires.

A man breaks an arm. He's back on the task at hand ten weeks later. The doctor cautions, "be careful, it's a new heal. It's sensitive. It could fracture again."

But he will also mention: once healed, the fracture will be stronger than the bone was originally.

Try to avoid those places, people, and stress situations which caused or cause you to repeat any episodes similar to the original ones you were prone to. I suggest you track these with a "journal of introspection."

I have a journal, which, like Band-Aids, is readily available to blot my wounds. It is always carried around, free, a source of self-check, but a great deal of the written sheets contain nothing but debris or the products of stress or reaction.

It's my ventilator system, so to speak. It also records my conversations, debts, remarks of my children or little genius utterances. I read it back to myself frequently. Daily, I cross out delusions, inaccuracies, or wrong observations, and I mark them as such. By doing this I so monitor myself.

Objectivity is my goal.

I pursue new items--I make pivotal behavior plans to nurse me through a trying confrontation.

I use it to face my own slipping back, or to deal with the consequences of my own behaviors.

Some of it is private, encoded to past moments or memories. So, for example, I may plan an exercise session to deal with exam stress while at school.

But, it could be tossed away today--I would not miss its contents. I am not dependent on it. It contains nothing I must remember. It is not indispensable.

I originally learned this technique at an experimental college as a form of descriptive writing or sociological recording--similar to Margaret Mead's notebooks in the field. We had to submit it to the college counselor along with our academic portfolio.

Over the years, I have adapted this tool to serve as my therapeutic outlet, besides my paintings, poems and novels. It works like a charm! Introspection and creativity walk hand in hand.   My suggestion to you: <u>borrow this tool</u>.

It will help you develop self-control.   You will know yourself better.   You must become your best friend and advocate.

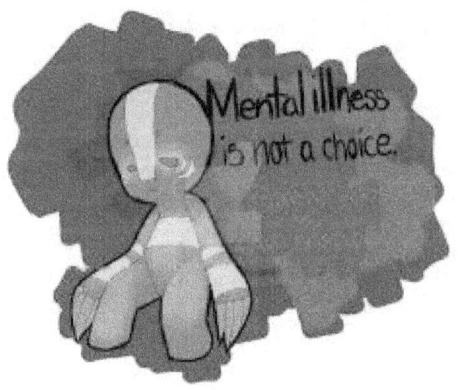

Chapter 5: Fountains, The Learning Path

I wanted to say a word about something useful to do when you are exploring yourself and seeking rehabilitation.

Did you come through a divorce, or did relatives abandon you in a town, without moorings? This may have been due to your confinement or natural circumstance. To tell the truth, many mentally ill people grapple with "shunning", or rejection by family and loved ones. They deal with the lack of a "life net" or the love and care provided by loved ones. This hinders recovery.

To find a springboard or place of recovery, do the following: you might benefit most by placing yourself back into the situation you were in when you were younger.

For example, return to your home town.

Did your health break while at college? Return to it! Register at the school.

Were you last in a city, at a career? Go to that familiar city.

Recently, without ready means to start over after divorce, both emotionally and economically, I returned to college. And I was already in my forties! I had been married, raised young children, and been divorced.

I never imagined the benefits of doing so--they were considerable! I can only attribute this to being constantly surrounded by younger and healthier people. In a sense, I returned to my own younger attitude. My spirit soared!

A college is sheltered. It can be more insulated, liberating and tolerant than, say, a factory town.

With respect to rules for older transfer students, l suggest that, initially, you rent a room in a home nearby and try a course, maybe not even for academic credit. You will find there are many helpers to get old academic records transferred.   And there well might be funding in the form of Federal student loans that you may be entitled to as, say, a war veteran.

After you begin classes, observe in yourself, the loss of intellectual and emotional "scars"! Shake off those wasted years! Give your intellect, your power of reason a "dust off".   Learn how to read and write once more. Force yourself to give an oral presentation before a group of sympathetic strangers.

You will awaken many sleeping social skills. You might go to a college football game with an acquaintance one weekend.   Time in the library is well spent. There is the latest technology and free computer equipment.   The media room is well stocked with movies and music CDs. There are clubs and organizations to join.   The Student Union is a stimulating place to meet new friends and enjoy leisure.

You will find, as I did, an incredible new bounce in your tread. With effort, you will brush up your old skills. You will shuck off years of negligence.

Rerouting your life when you are without roots is never easy.

A woman coming out of a divorce, where she lost all, will find, after a fruitless and insulting search through public agencies, this may be the <u>only viable springboard with the promise of a new future</u>.

Yes, colleges are a tremendous spring of vitality. Used with respect and humility, they will lead you to find and rebuild your identity again. Once strengthened, you will be able to choose a new direction or pick a new goal.

So, quickly leave what you must "back there", walk forward calmly, and build on your own youthful <u>persona</u>.   Your creative talents, in the college setting, will become active.

In the next semester, after preliminary exploration, apply for student housing.   At your age—you will be permitted to reside in a dormitory.   Ask for a solo studio.   There you will be, befriended by new dorm mates.   It will lift you up on wings of younger ideas and visions. Reclaim earlier dreams.   Find a job on campus, with work-study.   With meager earnings, purchase yourself a used car.

It is important that you place yourself in such a challenging position now.

A friend of mine, Peter, speaking in reference to a divorce with its results, suggested that the kids should be left to fend for themselves by both parents. "Let them sink or swim!" he said. I recall at the time I found the advice horrifying to consider. In the case mentioned, the kids did well when left on their own. They did visit me on campus on weekends.

Actually, it was sound advice. <u>Recovery requires being solo</u>, to face hard knocks, many tests, and harder challenges you will weather successfully.

With the adult finally out of talk therapy, it's hard to say "'try to stretch yourself" or "take a few more risks" knowing what that implies. The original conflict or engrained problem may rear its ugly head once more.

But it's any feared situation that you must face. Phobic insecurities cling to a healing personality. These tests of self-- shake loose the tight psychological muscles.

The results, with a series of small steps, can build you up, make you feel wonderful, and strengthen you. You feel like a gladiator who TKO's in the 3rd round.

Of course, sticking your neck out emotionally and being hurt by someone else is real pain. Of course, some of the knocks are being earned by an outdated attitude, or by psychologically-rooted lapses you are making, regrettably.

You should realize by now--that's a part of the daily role of being a complete adult.

One of the largest adjustments I made recently was feeling happy and loved, in situations that were previously socially poisonous.

Having high regard for yourself, based on the Lord's love for you, arises from a deep belief in your own solid moorings, your own future ahead, your strengths and integrity--as well as achievements and talents you carry as an individual. It is sensed by all meeting you. That makes you new friends and admirers.

Whatever dangerous situation or risky encounter, whether it be authoritarian or not, with an unshakeable hope in your heart--you are going to find the difficulties you imagined just evaporate.

I must say it's found to be a solid part of the Christian faith as expressed in the Eucharistic Mass in the saying "...with joyful hope, we await the coming..." It's an attitude for facing a bright new future along with the Redeemer. But in daily life for now, the attitude is an obligation on your part to be anxiety-free, to be peaceful. It's a new mindset, very desirable for you. Valid. Integrated.

"I give you peace. My peace I give you. Look not on our sins..." Jesus Christ said. This is worthy of meditation on your part. To leave those mental scars, bad memories, apprehensions, intolerant people behind with a buoyant smile, moving forward. What a titanic survivor you become! Others derive strength and serenity from you. This--I have seen with my own eyes. Quite the victory over Self!

I hope this message is clear even to the Moslem, Jew or pagan among us. You must shuck off the sick attitude of the mental patient and have hope in your heart as you take risks at a college. Whatever you've derived from therapy will be incorporated in your striving. You will be rehabilitating yourself in invigorating and safe waters. This path will lead you to a personal victory over the mental illness.

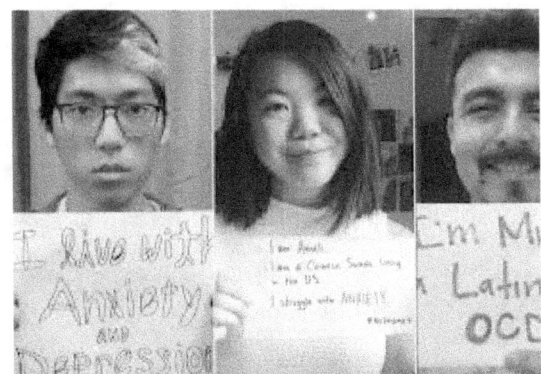 **I am working on it!**

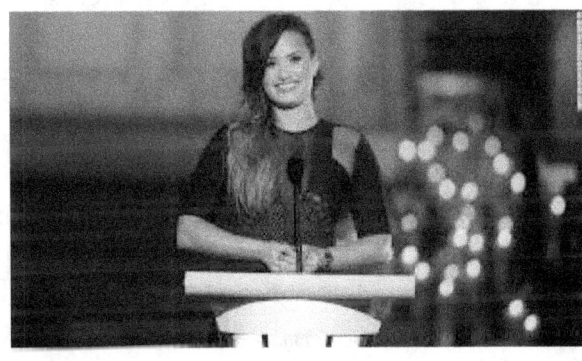 **I have overcome it!**

Chapter 6: Fortress

A person must view himself as a fortress and fortify inside. With each year, you add the stores of knowledge. You grow up with this, thinking, as you cultivate your hobbies, play sports, or read your books, that this all will mean little--but it means, later on, you have all this wealth of ideas to draw on and these, in very practical terms, give you strength.

In fact, the educated person will win hands down in any rehabilitation program. You just have a lot to use to succeed.

A recent British sit-com "Sherlock" developed the idea that one of its villains, paralleling Sherlock Holmes, had a "mind palace". To enter it, one had to close his eyes and deeply concentrate or meditate. Pretending to walk into the "mind palace", the character traversed hallways, climbed down staircases and found room after room, all memorized, of items he wished to remember. Opening a file drawer, he might retrieve a scribbled note or photograph he had as an eidetic image-- memorized, which was just the thing he needed[1]. Then, finished, he'd reverse his path up to the front door, close and lock it, and return to consciousness of his surroundings.

Each one of us is a "mind palace". We have entire rooms of knowledge, books, images, and any numbers of useful things we've learned in the past. The bigger the fortress or palace, the more stuff we have to find our talents and strengths in.

If you read Part Two, there's a posting about "Tony Steel Helmet". He was a counselor at a warm help line run by my home city for free. Tony was usually there if I dialed "211" on the phone. The thing about Tony was his strength. The guy had a steel helmet on in a metaphorical way of speaking. Nothing perturbed him. He was sure of himself, strong mentally, and had concrete views about most things. If you hit him with a current delusion, he deflected it for you. If you told him about your extreme pain and grief, he was cool, non-judgmental and hardly sympathetic. He had a lot of experience under his belt, had seen a lot of life. Perhaps he had been in the armed forces, or was a family man. He never divulged his personal life to me. The man lived life like a rhino. I began to copy him in mental stance and just grew and grew.

I would say, anyone with a lot of grit and experience, who has already been in a few marriages, say, or traveled a good deal, is going to be more resilient. That type of personality is an ideal role model for you.

It shows, not in how you take pressure, or how you handle a disturbing rejection. You might have a lot of education but be an emotional dunce.

You've got to go the distance. When you hardscrabble, you haul yourself in with a lot of the underpinnings you have. If it's a hobby you go back to that cradles you, why not? If it's sports that eases you through pain, good. If it's a new professor in a real estate certificate program that goads you into releasing your energies in a big new way-_-it's going to show.

So, in a sense, you never lose the debris, the time you invested earlier, or all those days and years--plus all the books, maps, charts, or the museum visits. Or the divorces, the miscarriages. You are enriched just the same.

And you should add to it. You should be a lifetime learner, developing your interests and talents as you grow older.

The stereotype of the mentally ill person is of a hyper-sensitive, flaky and strange "lone wolf". This person might become violent and explode. There's also the goofy, mindless and heavily drugged chain-smoker. Another portrait might be of an easily pressured person liable to mouth off all sorts of fantasies and delusions when barely provoked.

If you develop a fortress mentality, your self-control will increase. Less will bother you. And that's exactly the right stance to take when mingling with your fellow human beings.

Footnote:

[1]These are the abilities associated with **eidetic imagery**, more commonly known as photographic memory. **Eidetic imagery** has been defined as "the ability to retain an accurate, detailed visual **image** of a complex scene or pattern... or see an **image** that is an exact copy of the original sensory experience"

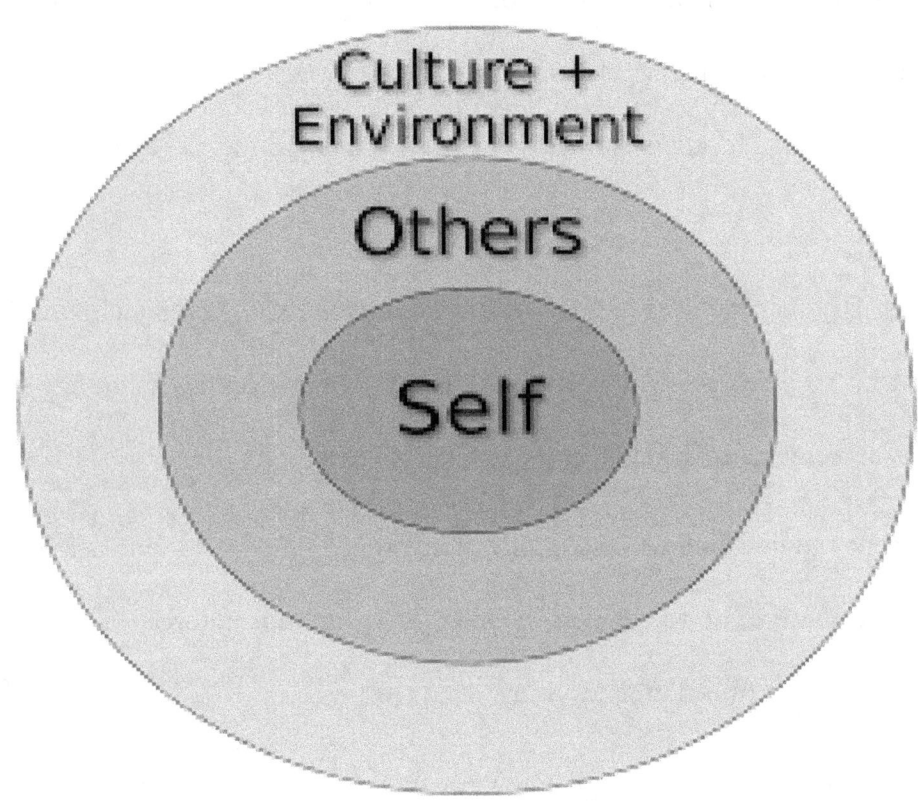

Chapter 7: Novelty

When you've had a lot of illness in your life, whether physical or mental, you tend to get psychologically constipated or streamlined in your lifestyle. You tend not to go into details, or take the time you might for the pleasant little interludes. Why? Partly, it's a feeling you missed out on something while you were hospitalized, so you've got to make up for lost time. The other reason is that you have become a coward. That's right!

With an "in treatment" lifestyle, you get more self-centered. You don't get into risky situations for many reasons. Gray places, ambiguous relationships--you don't wish to explore, because you might slip up, or you might get in too deep, or you might be wasting precious time. Even more possible, you'd be repeating the past. You'd be making the same social mistakes again.

Autism Spectrum Disorder includes extreme withdrawal, along with completely unsociable interactions with others. To a degree—you're mimicking that. No one yet has a cure for autism. But you can find one in recuperation from a chronic mental illness!

You have an urgency to live built up inside. The "can't waste time" syndrome is a habit--so break it! Forget who you were, or where you've been. Start with an enforced adjustment to leisure: make yourself relax for fifteen minutes a day. That's all!

Then, do something impulsive! Dine out at a new restaurant you pass on the road.

Proceed to flirting exercises once a week. Are you still too scared to try to pick up a good-looking man or woman? Step one--try a classified ad, or interact on an Internet dating website. There are myriad possibilities. All you have to do at first is want to try.

Seriously! These earned intense moments or new and intimate interactions are practice for your stultified feelings. Suspended animation, or being autistic, grants a stiffness like a mannequin. You need to thaw out and start feeling in the moment again.

Only seen your devoted mother for twenty-five years? Don't wait for any invitation! Step out into an openness in relationships. Go to a party, ask someone to dance, and leave the internal cage.

Hard to do! This doesn't happen overnight. Many recuperating people don't realize they stopped practicing a lot of social skills and facing day-to-day concerns in their mental illness war. And I'd like to prove to you why that richness day-to-day is necessary! Yes, "junk food, junk moments, and junk mail"—Don't judge yourself! Just_ dive in. Inhale. Flex. Inept social skills must be improved on. Thaw in. Feel new bursts of energy coming in from those around you. Try fourth gear inside. Try overdrive in the mental car. Can you trust yourself at a cocktail party? Can you ask for a new raise on the job?

One motion a day. Anything novel. Novelty tasks should rule.

The more, the better, like vitamins.

Middle-aged people are looking for this new air, by nature, anyway. It will feel like you're breathing pure oxygen when you start to try new behaviors.

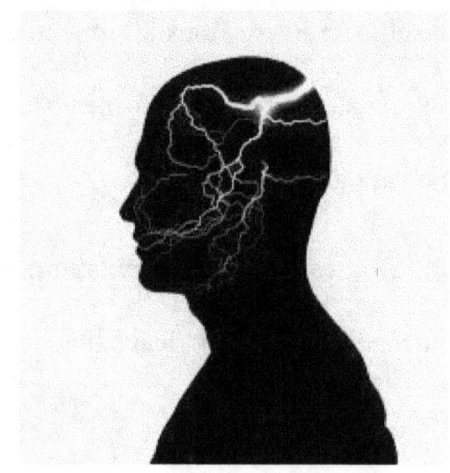

Chapter 8: Let Go

One big step I took toward health--a change of mindset--was a training of will I had to submit to. I trained myself to decide, to be decisive. Once I decided something, I "stuck to my guns", no matter what.

This simple resolve was initially tedious, painful, and against my nature.

Success practicing it has changed my life astonishingly to a large degree—making just this simple adjustment!

First--I am well-liked by such people as my children, because my word is my word. They have a firm personality to tussle with, and they model on me, perceiving decisiveness as strength.

The second change was to simply forget what the process was like, all the related weighing factors, memories, dialogues, lists, or other means I used to decide, or the intermediate steps I had taken to get there.

In other words, whatever part of my life I let go of, I really let go—and became oblivious to the indecisiveness which reigned before. I did not return to that decision. My personal life has become streamlined, as it were.

One sign of this is my progression of address books, showing the social decisions I have made over these months. I drop the contacts I decide are not friends. There are new ones, based on my decision to head toward new goals, or have new friends or circles of new ones.

Another sign is: If I have an argument or disagreement where I clearly have decided to "forgive and forget"-- I streamline my heart and mind in the way I thereafter walk through.... no arguments, trials, nothing like angry phone calls are made in an attempt to salvage what's gone. Simply, a line has been drawn, not to be crossed.   I know it, and accept fully that I must go on.

I accept my failures at friendship. Perhaps I turn the other cheek, like a Christian, and I feel a deep chagrin for a week. Perhaps the decision made is to extend a not in_ character apology. After, the slate is clean... we begin again on whatever new footing is socially expected. I forget and forgive whatever was before.

Believe it or not, an idea was derived from reading New Testament scripture.

Here is the pertinent passage:

(It starts in the Gospel of Mark, Chapter 9, Verse 43-45) *"If your hand causes you to sin, cut it off. It is better for you to enter life maimed, than to go into hell with two hands, where the fires never go out--.And if your foot causes you to stumble, cut it off.   It is better for you to entire life crippled than to be thrown into hell with two feet."* [2]

It became an experiment for me.

My motive was survival at first. A decision to cast off that sick part of me fighting my divorce is one example.   There were deep feelings of grief, outrage and conflict. One streamlining effect, since I "let go", in very practical terms, was the efficiency of my academic life afterward at a university, where I was better able to concentrate quietly on learning for hours. My grades rose noticeably and I ended up earning two degrees afterward, graduating "summa cum laud" (with highest honors).   I wish my dear mom could have lived to see that day, the day when her "sick kid" became a capped and gowned Masters student.

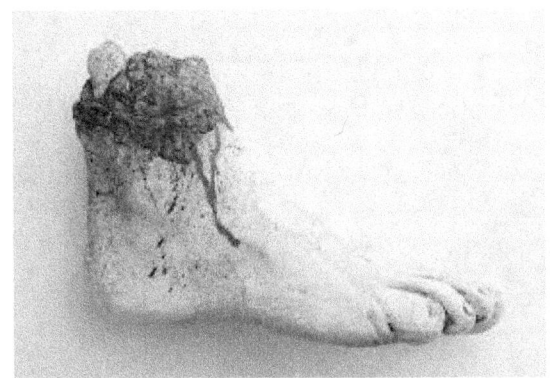

Footnotes:

²paraphrased from the Bible, New International Version.

Chapter 9: Design Your Schedule

In keeping with the idea that patience is key to recovery, I note here that I have proof in my own story. I designed a new lifestyle to meet new goals. I strove to shuck off the mental illness. This, while living in poverty with an aging parent!

Although emotionally sick from a divorce, I proceeded to maximize my situation coolly and practically. True, I had been dealt a blow in the loss of child custody. I thought it through, coming up with a design which fit my psychological needs and concrete facts.

I could perhaps return to school—with financial aid. Indeed, I wanted to finish my degree. I applied to several colleges and asked for student loans. I decided to live on campus in a dormitory. That would be nice, although I would be mingling with students twenty-five years younger than myself. It was allowed!

Almost by accident, I worked my way into a brand new situation which was very beneficial to me. First of all, I got away from my past--family and any places which made me sick or sad. The new life's focus was narrow, and there were few distractions. There were no new emotional triggers for delusions, and I was once again independent. Nor were there demanding activities from a full-time job. I was at college once more, and happy about it. For the time being, I was financially secure. I felt younger immediately—never a bad thing.

Now my weekday schedule was very regular. I scheduled my courses to allow me to rise in the late morning. There was more than enough leisure to rest my weary soul. Travel was not a big problem either.

I had little conflict left in my personal life. There were no demanding relationships, although I still visited my emotionally-needy children on weekends. That was my main stress.

My achievement in the study of psychology was more than I might have expected at the age of 45.   I had narrowed my focus to finish something I had begun twenty years ago. I succeeded in attaining "A"s, and making the Dean's List.

But notice this: I did now have a mental illness. There was the start of auditory hallucinations after a head injury. So, I spent a disproportionate time reading, preparing, and backtracking through review.

I really had no other distractions, far less than most other people.   *I needed quiet and solitary hours, more than most.* There was a lot of ease and rest time built in to an essentially undemanding, but full day. For example, on Monday, Wednesday, and Friday my schedule allowed me, after noon, to pursue my hobbies. These included swimming, taking walks, and reading.

Designing the lifestyle was a real breakthrough.   You may have to go to such lengths to get on track to recovery.

After academic achievement arrived, my increased self-esteem itself became my springboard.   It intensified my desire to achieve self-improvement in other areas. For example, I found it possible to enjoy my involvement with my children with less angst. I brought them to stay-overs on campus.   I met with some new friends from time to time. I even tried going to dating socials.   Swimming often was a solid attempt to start a new weight loss regimen. It was also a great stress reducer.

I had a much higher level of confidence to be applied here. I directed it to deal with any leftover problems from the past which remained.

It is apparent that, to recover and develop yourself in the most straightforward and healthy fashion, you must design into your day-to-day schedule the greatest amount of opportunity for extra time and comfort, or "pampering", to compensate for your mental frailties or internal emotional obstacles.   My dear, you are damaged.

With that design, *which you must not construe as selfish, greedy, self-seeking, or self-centered*, you will see what unfolds--a great surprise, most rewarding.   It will be a return of mental health and youthfulness!

With the design of a new lifestyle, your chances of success in curing yourself will be markedly increased.

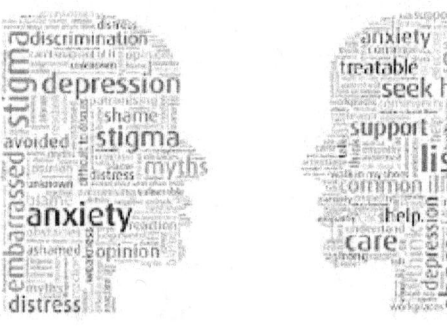

Chapter 10: Alienation-- How To Keep The Home Fires Burning

Most people, whether sick or well, aren't built to be alone for long periods. I doubt those who do are very fulfilled. You want to be with people.

Feeling cut off socially is also internal. Spores last through Winter, rough neighborhoods, and heavy change, but flower only in the right conducive environment.

Be a cactus flower, a bit prickly, but when there's some moisture, by all means, reach out.

I compare social mixing to body surfing in high, heavy surf. When those swells come in, dive under, bounce over the slights, rejections, or the coolness. When the right person comes along, catch the tempo of the dialogue, enjoy, and ride the wave in--go with it!

Know your limits. Don't become stubborn and try to force yourself on others, standing there getting buffeted, slammed by each crest. With bending and avoiding undertows, some pretty decent conversation can be had. Savor that. <u>Just don't expect commitment or deep involvement.</u>

My therapist once told me that it takes seven years, on average, when relocating to a new town, to make real friends. It's a slow process of trust and exploration.

There is a stigma to being mentally ill. People gossip. There may be a conscious effort by a prejudiced individual to spread it around about you. As a former neighbor, an acquaintance, or a friend of a friend, he might just know your diagnosis. He feels it's his civic duty to warn people away. This is hard to take, for often you have already been shunned by relatives. So you are wearing a label, wherever you go.

I chose to break with my past and joined a church in a new town. Within a month or two, a well-meaning priest had gained full knowledge of my mental infirmity from my confession, in confidence. He dealt with it by broaching the subject of mental illness with his congregants. All of a sudden, the church people were being told to love their mentally ill brethren.   An outside deacon whose ministry was to serve the inmates of a local psychiatric hospital and prison came to speak on the presence of the mentally ill there, how to spot them, and how to interact with them.   My priest even asked, at one point, for members of the church who were mentally ill or had a mentally ill family member to raise their hands, be counted, and "loved".

All of this made me quite uneasy.   I felt like I was walking in a spotlight all the time. Several new acquaintances shunned me.   People knew I was "one of those" and did not befriend me.   Things were on a pretty superficial level for years afterward.   It ruined my expectations for leaving my past behind.   And, of course, the parson who had broken confidence with me— no longer could be trusted with anything spiritual.   He had done something morally wrong.

You will be forced to deal with shunning and prejudice.   You will be labeled and bear the stigma of the social misfit. Just remember one thing--you have to keep your own lamp lit. You can't run away, nor can you avoid facing others despite their knowledge of your "affliction". For goodness sakes, don't lose your faith in the Lord over it.   Yes, you will be sorely tried. Keep the faith!

Walk out into the waters of life and dive in!   Socialize to save your psyche.   Keep trying with new people.   This will aid your recovery immeasurably.

Mental Illness
is not
Contagious

You Can't Catch it
by Being Kind

What if your insurance company treated your cancer diagnosis the same way they treated your mental illness?

Chapter 11: A Word on Fatigue

Recovery is best achieved, as mentioned before, if you optimize that which produces health. And in this case, it's *rest*.

When you have had a particularly long and difficult day where, temporarily, you've been forced to make a serious life-or-death decision or judgment, or been forced to perceive a lot of novel things about your life all at once--there is present a real danger.

This is your enemy called *mental fatigue*.

First of all, become aware of your own cycles. Maybe, like myself, you are going to be most clearheaded, fresh, and stable on mornings, during those first few hours. Take advantage of this self-knowledge to do more then.

Remember, after periods of strain as mentioned above--where you have a clear case of mental exhaustion--your new psyche is going to be penetrable like your skin. Given the wrong incident, such as a violent and unbalancing dialogue with verbal spears cast at you, you are highly vulnerable to a return to a symptomatic state.

This is all due to mental fatigue: tics, depressive inaction, delusion-filled schemes--whatever your diagnosis description initially was, for better or worse, whether you believe it was on the mark or not, it may show up again when you open your mouth. Psychological illness doesn't happen like colds--but a fatiguing day allows your lapses to cause trouble eventually. I find, with more mental gymnastics, your mentality folds responsively, even more quickly than your immune system. Depression, minor allergies, or the huge number of decisions you need to make can increase the speed of onset for this moment of crisis.

A rationale to continue along the wrong course of action is deadly. Pulling in the reins on your own tired tendencies must result when you first recognize in yourself what is happening.

Pull out that journal you're keeping and examine what's written there! You either seek to minimize these days and prevent their ever happening, or you submit to actual self-training to spot the root symptoms you display early, with a good mirror, before disorder really starts to happen!

There is a limit to any tool kit you use. Sick thinking comes with its own autonomy, with a compulsion inside to give in to it, or to repeat. Almost like a wild beast within you, it desires to exist, to operate its own wheels. Resisting this compulsion which drives maladjustment is difficult.

When that day happens, remember the myth of the Sirens and Theseus: strap yourself to your mast, fill your ears with wax, and let the little boat sail past where the delusions sing. You will survive.

In more practical terms, halt it in any way possible. For example, whatever you are doing, pause--back up! Is it driven by emotion? I suggest that you switch your environment, get away, and do some physical chore. Try watching a Bogart movie. Don't let the bad state stay. Don't allow it to last for more than that one day. Episodic breaks railroaded by a demanding mental situation? Seek the help of a counselor.

But, to halt it when it begins—first remove fatigue. Correct! Cancel all appointments, lock the door, and, if required, administer a reliable headache breaker like aspirin. Take a hot shower, put on your "fuzzy-wuzzie" slippers, and, after a glass of warm milk, set your alarm for at least ten hours later, before you dive under the covers. Look in the mirror. Say, "I forgive you. I love you." Go to sleep. Sleep that fatigue away.

You may not need to do anything more.

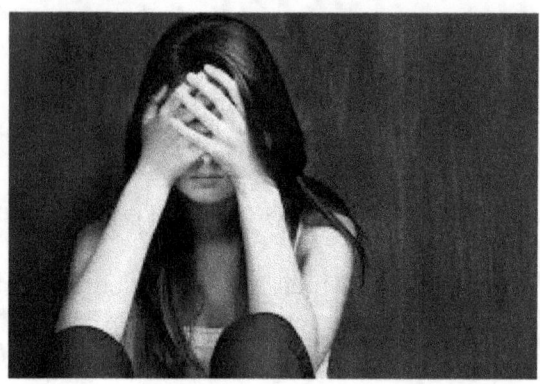

Chapter 12: The Schedule

I have lived in two different and extreme lifestyles. The first one was having employment and attending school courses which dictated what I did every minute of a weekday.

In the second case, I was involved with no schedule: no watch, no clocks, and a day of unrestricted freedom and liberty!   Can you deal with that? Or, rather, are you afraid, like most who recover, that you will slip into the twilight zone of indecision or daydream, delusion-filled, that you used to dwell in?   It is waiting just around the next corner, right?

Well—don't panic! Keep in mind that a lot of contribution to your state of mind was a security blanket-type insulation provided to you by your friendly pharmacist and doctor. It put you into a coddled fog.

Now, recovered, you would be chemically free. But yes—you're prone to a relapse.

So settle into a daily routine of self-directed chores which you divide between keeping yourself engaged with life and doing physical labor.

Watch the fear of no schedules ebb away! You will eventually feel comfortable with action at will. Yes, basically, you will enjoy the freedom even while hesitation, or "waffling" and indecision will be lightly repeated. It takes time. Be patient. Failing is no crime.

At the other extreme--the high pressure schedule with no control--you have forty projects with deadlines to complete way too soon.   You might have become, for example, an art director who is still on job probation.   Perhaps you now have an impossible boss. You should have some ideas to aid you in self-control.

You must have some sense something is wrong when you schedule too much because you fatigue and mess up. You must get this across to the manager in any job situation you enter. Your boss has to be an understanding and good person, too. Deliberately find one like that!

By trying a gradual climb, or a moderate schedule of work for the day, and by controlling your own workload, you will allow yourself to succeed. You might do better as a movie usher, rather than a fast-food restaurant counter person.

Here's a proposed method to schedule if you're a student. It could be adapted to being a company employee:

Each morning, I resort to my address book and calendar book to plan the day. On my index cards are the list of must do's, can do's, should do's, like-to-do's, and love-to_-do's.

I start, then, with priority numbers. Musts get a one, shoulds are the twos, and any others I will try to do are threes. This little card is referred to. I stick it in my back pocket, back it up with a copy I leave at home, pack my book bag, collect the mail, the keys, check the spare change-- and I'm out the door. All of this leaves me clear_ headed and prepared for a relatively structured day.

You could easily use an app on your tablet or Smart phone to do this.

But, I recommend that you, to get to a "permanent health zone", do what I did—on a weekend, go for a retreat and spend a couple of "different days", sans watches or shoes. Try meditation, a Circle of Mary, or go to *shul* on Saturday morning! These are the times your soul centers in complete security. You can achieve a confident liberty while living in free, unstructured time. This is what I would recommend you do. Begin to trust yourself.

You need to have both types of schedule.   There should be days where you're totally free and liberated from work and study demands, where you're stable and having a pleasant time. Your scheduled and structured days should be relaxed enough to allow you to remain balanced and productive.   You be the judge.   You design it to empower you to be well.

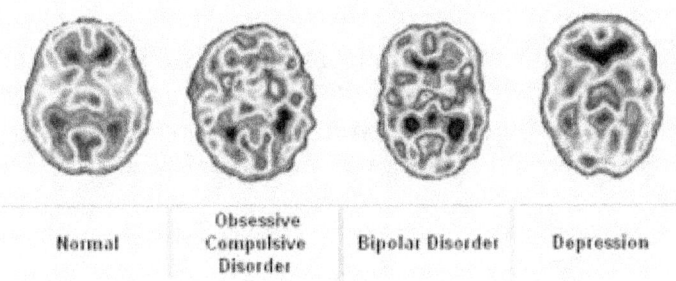

Normal   Obsessive Compulsive Disorder   Bipolar Disorder   Depression

Chapter 13: Built On A Rock

You must trust your basic relationships to your marriage partner, friends or children. You must rely on what you see as being exactly what it is, like you are a rock.

Fight delusions.

A friend recently suffered an anxiety attack based on pure doubt. A delusion about his son took hold, he acted out, and he wound up in the hospital for a week of needed treatment and medication. While taking a walk, he had seen the boy where there was nobody to be seen. It had made him frantic. He began to act out, chasing a car down the road. A car with a stranger inside!

Be strong. Don't doubt relationships.

Your anxiety attacks well may tear down the superstructure of a place to be, relationship, and normal routine in short order.

Keep strong. Be resolute. You--especially--are subject or vulnerable to the vicissitudes of your own mind going wrong.

If you have to--*get professional help fast*. See the psychiatrist you went to last year immediately. Don't be afraid. Just do it.

The penalties of being on the other side of reality can be earth shattering. You just dissolve as a personality.

Above all--be adamant when you decide what's what is reality.

REALITY? HMMM.

Chapter 14: Love Yourself

After a setback, placed in favorable circumstances, I found myself at many moments having time for idle reflection. "Wasted time" or "treats" or "whatever I wish activity" filled some hours. After pleasure, there was tangible guilt.

However, these moments were a kindness I paid myself. They were investments I made in myself. My attractiveness and my need to seek male companionship pulled me down a road to new activities. What I felt was chagrin that it was so necessary.

Afterward, when good feelings and tranquil spirit took hold as a result of doing these small things which were pleasant only to me, I knew I had found a new source of strength and resilience for myself.

What sort of things might these be? Here are some suggestions. You might have a "day of beauty or handsome", with a massage, a new hair style, or manicure. You could visit a museum for the day—the one with the pricey admission. You might try stepping out dressed up and go to a happy hour at your favorite neighborhood bar. You might take a paragliding lesson. The list is endless.

Since then, I seldom look back on the petty self-denier I was. I know that making myself well, strong, and vigorous encourages me and I reap health back. These indulgent pastimes are necessary for me to feel my worthiness and to become a successful person. I have the capacity to have new experiences and new feelings and then say: "I am now somebody".

I am sure this is what the doctors intend with all their therapy. You should encourage yourself to enjoy your own needs, hobbies, and company. Become your own friend, to your immense benefit.

Chapter 15: What Comes First

Before one can be safely out of the woods of mental illness, one must reach a new plateau of ego strength. That means, a strong, capable, and firm footing of some kind. You must reach a threshold of strength, and it only comes after tremendous effort. And it must take years.

I don't know what it will be for you. You may, like myself, take a risk and seek to become an "impossible" dream. It will require all your energies, new skills, and the strength (there's that word again) to see it through. In my case, it was finishing my college degree. I eventually had to prepare for tests, take them, and pass them.   I wanted to earn some kind of social recognition.

In so doing, you will have less and less moments of weakness. You will know who you are, in the full sense of the word. The achievement will be something no one can ever take away from you, once earned.   It will give you a new sense of pride.

Then, you won't have to hold on to that broken image of who you are, "the failure", "the nut job", or whatever pet names you called yourself.

When you have done this, you will be able to stretch and reach for other tangible signs of success as a human being—companionship, the love of friends, perhaps even, in time, a new partner.

So---pick a goal--a really hard one.

What the goal is is not as important as the process of getting there.

After you reach it, the phase of your life when you were suffering from mental illness will be firmly in the past.   It will have been placed behind you, where it belongs.

Our lives go through phases, after all.

Perhaps you will still carry a label like "bi-polar" or "obsessive-compulsive", but it will only be one small part of your life. You'll see someone for medication a few times a year, and chat, and that's all.

Inside, your trained mind will be still and strong. It will function well when you need it. Emotionally, there will be a tremendous reserve and a boost which help you face new challenges with assurance and surmount them easily.

I say this after doing it. And you must do it too.

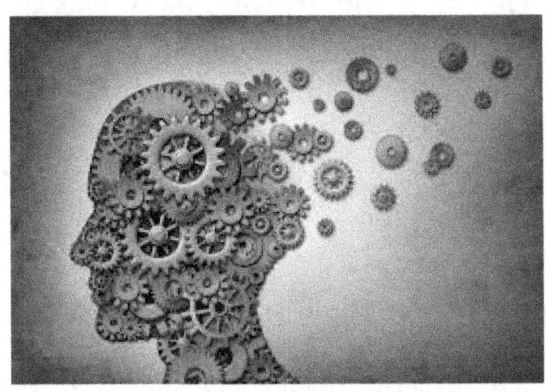

Chapter 16: Drastic Measures

It is necessary to employ drastic measures in the case where the aforementioned therapeutic methods have been insufficient to produce a full cure. The style of life has rendered the patient a precarious and fragile balance which will crumble under the pressures of a work schedule or social ostracism. Perhaps there has been an unusual series of crimes committed against society or oneself, producing trauma as a steady diet and psychological scars.

There is one overwhelming thought to hold in place: a return to happiness is imperative, and can occur. Never consider yourself beaten in finding a way to cure yourself.

It may be best after enduring the adverse conditions or a relapse into your particular diagnosis to take a vacation. By doing so, you can juxtapose the usual and the novelty of the new country or locale. If you are indeed able to function happily on tour, you have proven scientifically that at home there are stresses masked or revealed which are precipitating a mental illness impacting on your life. It might be displayed as paranoia, insomnia, or the symptoms of your unique diagnosis.

If such is the case even after being in Britain or Japan, consider relocating permanently to cure yourself. This in itself is a highly stressful choice of therapy. As mentioned above, one must never lose one's optimism regarding an eventual return to a healthful adjustment to life. Be brave enough to find a new home which will in turn eventually cure you.

A word of caution: chronic chemical imbalances of the neurotransmitters in your brain might be entrenched, and although they may gradually subside, it might take long months to see a positive impact. But I affirm that this will come.

So, start! Begin by researching likely places for that transfer. Go on the Web and relive the vacation, choosing a closer place within your budget. There will be a need to pay a mover or public storage. You might have to put a house up for sale. These things take time to do properly.

A middle step might be to simply pack a suitcase, and during a series of long weekends, travel to desirable cities or towns you might wish to explore. Spending very little, go during weekdays when local Chambers of Commerce and realtors are open for business. Rental cars or public buses will take you around. Look at the beaches and parks. What sort of gyms or recreational programs are available? What is the cost of living compared to your former town? Take good notes and ask pedestrians questions. Finally, make a checklist of pros and cons as you return home. If there are few benefits, wait a week or two and venture somewhere else.

This writer decided in April, 2009 to find a town where she might find work, live reasonably well, avoid traffic and congestion, and enjoy a country setting. In June, packing only one suitcase and reserving a cheap room in a private home through a popular website (craigslist.com), she traveled by bus to that city and took up residence. In the weeks ahead, setting up a temporary mailbox, she explored the city stem to stern.

There were many things pleasant and wonderful about the new town. For one thing, people were friendly and polite, greeting strangers in the morning with a hello. The price of food and lodgings was over 25% cheaper than at home. Additionally, the city held many festivals, had a high functioning group of social service agencies, and gave her a feeling of well-being with its beautiful scenery along a river. Venturing to apply at an apartment house for those over 55, she was overjoyed to be accepted. With Fall approaching, she was forced to make a decision as she returned to her former home.

The writer had been harassed for over a year by some unknown criminals. She had made over 10 police reports of suspicious incidents or petty larcenies at her apartment. And she suspected a former spouse or neighbor as the culprit. She decided that she wanted to break all family ties permanently. Her siblings had made her life miserable for years. She consulted with a former F.B.I. agent, seeking to gain anonymity and protection under the law. He advised her to relocate and obtain a new legal name. So she visited the County Clerk's Office.

Truly, there was a feeling of hope in her heart and healthy plans for the future. She would need to retrieve her belongings from public storage later, but she could pick up a suitcase or two more. Adding a bicycle and some kitchen items, finishing up some legal proceedings which required her presence, and transferring her mailbox and bank account took up a week or so. Then, armed with a new legal name, the patient once again took a bus to her new home.

At first it was very stressful and she had a return of symptoms. But within a month, she had received generous support in the form of Medicare, Medicaid, Food Stamps and SSDI. It enabled her to beautifully furnish her new home, settle all debts, and begin a new life in relative comfort.

Joining a local church, she became active as a member and, within a year, had over fifty new acquaintances. To her delight, there was no privation being without a car as the new town had an outstanding public bus system. She joined the local college's fitness center to mix and mingle with young people. As mentioned in an earlier chapter, colleges can be a "fountain of youth".

Particularly urgent was settling into a new therapeutic relationship. A talk therapist, a psychiatrist, and an outstanding hospital found later--our patient was all set. The year which followed found her making good progress in addressing entrenched psychological problems.   A local wellness center had a support group with free group therapy once a week.

All in all, after a year, she found a doctor to suit her needs who was skillful in prescribing a new medication for her mental condition.   Lo and behold, it was remarkable in the way it removed her symptoms, enabled her to sleep and become more adjusted and flexible.

There is always a positive solution to medically improve yourself.   Simply finding a new therapist or prescription might be the answer. (Although, it is certain that frequent change of a doctor is a sign that you have a problem which is resisting likely steps to success.)

The above case is but one personal and somewhat extreme example.

Change of scenery, a change of name, or a change of lifestyle far away from the people who hurt you, or the job that was impossible, or the landlord who was making life expensive might switch the mental illness off, just like that temporary fix of a trip to another country.   It could be advantageous to leave your parents, siblings, and former significant other behind. Those were dysfunctional relationships.   They should be discarded like debris.

Additionally, you must assume there is a city or town out there which is superior to your hometown. It might have a beautiful spectrum of services and agencies tailored to bring you quick relief and support for your handicap.

Most important is your mindset and resiliency.   Take the risk of relocating to a better fit for you.   The tool kit you battle mental illness with will be bigger, sturdier and more ingenious.

What is the lesson here?   Never give up or assume after years of effort that there is no solution around the next corner.   You have applied all the techniques described in this book and the showdown has not ended.   That does not mean you have done something wrong--FOR IT

WILL NEVER END.

But--you will know you are going to win soon enough. THEN YOU WILL!

Part One: Conclusion-

A person who develops a mental illness has undergone a dramatic shift in brain chemistry which alters the personality and dynamic of the sufferer in telling ways. Were you to faithfully follow the program outlined in Part One of this book, you would gradually improve over a long course of time. That is my prediction, but there are exceptions to the rule in every case.

Having a Showdown With Mental Illness, begun around 1996, has now been completed over 19 years later. The course of my own mental illness has entered the recovery phase, and I consider my mental illness to be "in remission". My friend, it took *19 years* of struggle and hard work to reach my dream.

The brain is a remarkable "crown of creation" which is capable of recovery. It finds new ways to balance and neural pathways to utilize. Even so, the genetic predisposition to mental illness is still locked into the DNA code of your body.

Progress can be made to a remarkable degree.

Your future life free of mental illness will require constant vigilance, monitoring, use of a therapeutic tool kit, and adherence to a set of rules affecting your lifestyle. There will be daily decisions to make concerning activities. You will be forced to decide moment to moment to accept or deny a perception, a rumination, a delusion-filled daydream. As your self-awareness improves, the emergence of these symptoms will decrease.

In entering recovery, you will be a changed person. Don't be a fool and declare yourself cured. March on, faithfully following those new guidelines and practices which optimize your mental health. Yes, you will enjoy the remainder of your life.

PART TWO: PERTINENT TOPICS—IN RECOVERY

Introduction to Part Two, "The Blog"

When this book was originally conceived it had sixteen chapters outlining a program of simple steps one could follow to end a chronic mental illness. Nineteen years later, when on the other side of recovery, the author rewrote the book. Using hindsight and recollection, some of the ideas changed but the main steps of the program remained the same because it had been largely successful.

The greatest change was a misconception of time frame. In 1997, the author was certain that her program would lead to a cure within a couple of years. However, the entrenched nature of the author's mental illness was coupled with chronic dysfunction in primary relationships within her family unit. These worked against her over time to partially neutralize the positive effects of following this program. Good habits could not overcome the precariousness of homelessness, lack of acceptance and love, or opportunities for gainful employment.

After taking the most drastic step of reinventing herself (as outlined in Chapter 16 of Part One), the author succeeded in recovering from her chronic mental illness. However, once again, it must be mentioned that there were some residual effects.

But the tendency to have auditory hallucinations may have been the result of a series of head injuries over the years. Additionally, the unique biochemistry of the author, as a result of a traumatized case of acute childhood asthma in which repeated injections of epinephrine were administered, encouraged a remaining tendency to explode in manic stream-of-thought episodes when the "fight or flight" response was triggered by her environment.

What I am saying here is that you, the Reader, may have better results in achieving the total remission of your condition than I was.   That would be my guess.

To continue: after 19 years the author achieved a state of remission or significant cure. She was capable of reaching her personal goals.   She found happiness, contentment and fulfillment in her daily life.   It was more success than she could have ever hoped for.

However, as it developed, there were many "loose ends" or perceptions arising from a dramatic recovery which had not been incorporated in the first manuscript.   Part Two is an attempt to address this development.

In the course of three years, from 2013-2015, this author input over 47 blog posts on the wordpress.com website covering all sorts of topics pertinent to a mentally ill person in our society.

These have now been reviewed and sorted into several categories by subject matter.   Part Two contains the best of these.   It is designed as a resource for the recovering individual to enable understanding of the underpinnings and causes of mental illness in the prone party, the types of tools available in the community, and how to develop the best attitude toward yourself and others.

This blog, expanding and current, can be viewed at: marykhazakgrant.wordpress.com.

Chapter 17: General

Having a Showdown with Mental Illness (2014-09-09 19:54)

I am starting this blog to publish ideas on how to fight a schizophrenic condition based on my own direct experience.

I feel qualified because I am both a writer and a person having a showdown daily. All the successful methods I have devised in self-managed care will be included.

I am presently in recovery, having received approval this summer, 2014 to refrain from seeing a psychiatrist any further. For history, let me state that I have been mildly schizo-affective since 1972. That's right! Over 31 years.

That goes along with a bipolar axis. So, you readers suffering from that disorder will also find a lot of useful strategies and methods of control here as well.

Let me say that, despite my condition, I have become a high achiever. I am possessed with a Masters degree in education, one in which I graduated cum laud. I have a B.A. degree in Psychology as well. I also work as a teacher. As an author, I have self-published over 10 books.

So this blog may, from me to me, contain useful and inspiring ideas for budding authors.

But primarily, it will be devoted to "Having a Showdown with Mental Illness", introducing some novel new methods which lead to self-cure. I have been the guinea pig. Take advantage of my knowledge!

The Dangers of Drug Abuse Are Considerable (2014-09-30 13:50)

You are a zany, wild teenager dabbling in soft drug use. Your mind is your experimental tool, your door of discovery to new states of consciousness, delirious, distorted and imaginary.

What you do not know is that your gene code blueprint, the DNA code in your body, is disposed toward mental illness.

The sites turn on and off in your mind–and, as a result, your brain chemistry takes you for a prolonged ride into mental illness. It's something you can't switch off at will.

You stop abusing drugs, prescription or street. Despite that, you are forced to submit to episodes which mimic the drug trances. Sometimes you have visual hallucinations–pretty pink dots pass before your eyes. Maybe you see people on the sidewalk who vanish into thin air.

After a few months of enjoyment, you grow fearful. Your family checks you into a hospital for observation. You are tentatively diagnosed as a schizophrenic person with psychotic episodes.

This now is your reality. It all started because you abused drugs.

I suggest that if you recognize this portrait you cease and desist from taking medication which wasn't prescribed for a legitimate medical condition. Have yourself evaluated by a psychiatrist. Do it for your own survival.

I don't have handy the exact percentage figures regarding a genetic predisposition for mental illness. It's a fairly new field of research, less than 20 years old. People cannot yet be screened for the gene code flags. According to Dr. Lloyd I Sederer, M.D., author of The Family Guide to Mental Health Care (W.W. Norton & Co., 2013), one percent of the global population has schizophrenia. It's a safe bet that a larger percentage has some form of mental illness. By the way, this is an excellent book to start understanding what you and your family need to do when mental illness rears its ugly head in your life.

But to be more practical, it's as easy as walking in to your college advisor at your university, or visiting the guidance counselor at your high school, or having a talk with your family doctor. That's the best start.

The Role of Bored Solitude in Making Mental Illness (2015-06-25 19:06)

I have been alone for over twenty years since I divorced in 1995. For the bulk of the aftermath, I have been in bored solitude. It's conducive to mental illness. I want to document the impact of that social condition on the psyche of the individual seeking a cure. It's a steep uphill climb. Social obstacles are daunting.

As someone living on SSID, along with part time wage earnings, I make just enough to sustain a poor lifestyle. It's not just food clothing and shelter. You must pay for therapy and entertainment. There's little budgeting for pleasures possible. A person must in a sense buy friends. That is to say, you might meet some people at meet.up.com if you can spend on drinks at the bar, appetizers and fuel for your vehicle. That is, if you even have a vehicle. Having a car is one of the most significant walls to hurdle when poor. Some never manage it. Others are impoverished by the cost.

There is no guarantee that, should you go to local events and happenings, that you will meet a person seeking companionship.

My apartment house is populated by grotesques, freaks and people in extreme need. I do not mingle with them–they are, for the most part, incompatible to me. I have a developed intellect, I have college degrees and a professional certification. Not so my neighbors, all of whom are over fifty-five. Over sixty-five is even more common. This is not an oasis for socializing.

So you find that yes, you can manage to survive but you cannot afford outlets which lead to expense. And so–you end up sitting more and more in front of that great time waster: the television set.

Bored solitude produces a loss of sensitivity. The monotony may lead to excessive use of rituals, diaries, calendars or chat rooms. You're constantly thrown back on your own devices for amusement

I will develop this train of thought more later. It hurts me to have to write about it. I am so alone in the world at this point–I can go almost full days without speaking to another soul.

How to Become Psychotic Real Fast (2015-07-05 18:22)

This post will be a little tongue-in-cheek. If you want to see any recessive or precursive mentally ill traits manifest in your psyche, I have some suggestions for you. I speak from personal experience.

Here's my list:

1. Drink alcohol a lot. All times of day. Any me you're stressed. It will produce delusional, paranoid and hallucinatory symptoms galore–no time flat!

2. Do drugs. Soft/hard–your choice. They will completely screw up your nervous system. Drugs like LSD may cause a permanent change in your brain chemistry. You'll be seeing dots in front of your eyes at high stress moments ("rabbititis") and worse.

3. Practice Eastern mysticism or religion. With extreme asceticism and a meager vegetarian diet along with mindless chanting, spinning or focusing on the wall–any predisposition for mental illness will tend to manifest.

4. Immerse yourself in the occult–in writings and speculations of the great mystics. You are guaranteed to have your grip on normal reality loosened.

5. Mingle with Devil worshippers. Some very strange, bad things will happen to you. You will doubt your own perceptions, my friend. Guarantee it–you'll destabilize and go off the deep end.

Well, that's about it. Youth wants to know, is curious and experiments with all of the above. It can have a profoundly detrimental effect on your life, your health, and your dreams. As I told my son, do any of the above and you will lose ten years of your life wasted–more likely than not.

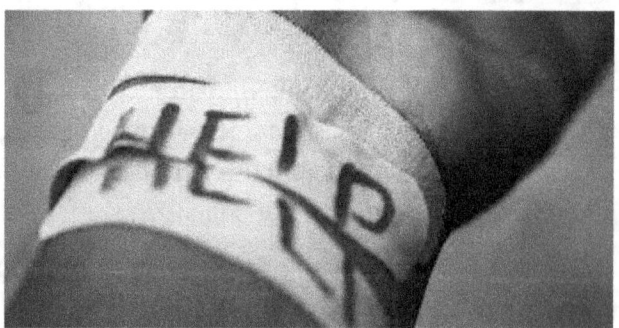

Chapter 18: TOOLKIT

Fighting Mental Illness with Meditation (2014-09-10 21:10)

The struggle in functioning well with a mental illness like my schizo-affective disorder may lead you down many strange roads–roads you would never have been on but for the inner drive to be made well. It led me at an early age to explore yoga in all its myriad forms and meditation.

Yoga is an ancient 5,000 year-old system of spiritual discipline. You may read about it in the writings of ancient Hindu sages such as *Shankara* or *Patanjali*. To study yoga best, read The Bhagavad-Gita. This describes the classic practice. For anyone seeking more than enlightenment, Yoga may be a framework for practices which lead to higher inner harmony in the body, perceptual enhancement and clarity, increased energy, and mental control.

Meditation can be practiced through various schools of discipline. You usually must sit in a quiet seated position on a pillow for some me. There are many sorts of meditation. TM, Transcendental Meditation was popularized by the Beatles in the 1960's. Yoga meditation utilizes techniques at the start of each session which involve pranayama or breathing exercises. This in itself is a great an dote to stress and tension. Another sort of meditation is Zen meditation,

which involves keeping your eyes open while you concentrate on the wall.

I practiced meditation for many years. It was beneficial. I suggest it as a powerful tool to decrease the misperceptions or delusional streams which flow through the mind of a mentally ill person. If you can simply become the observer, gazing at your own perceptions, feelings and thoughts as they constantly change without becoming enmeshed in them, you will develop a strength of psyche which will counteract the destabilizing tendencies of a mental condition such as schizophrenia. You can practice on or off medication. Usually, half an hour a day is enough to bring about a beneficial effect.

One word of warning. Do not practice Zen meditation if you have a mental illness. It is a well-known fact that zazen brings about hallucinations, both visual and auditory if you do it for long periods of me.

Meditation will relax and invigorate you. It will center your ego in a quiet objective state. Give it a try! Make it a habit!

Music as Therapy (2014-09-27 15:12)

What follows are some guidelines and suggestions to incorporate music into your "tool kit" to control mental illness.

I do not know how I could survive without music influencing my daily life. Whether I passively listen to it or make it, music acts like a tonic to mi gate the most outlandish or extreme hallucinations suffered with my schizophrenic disorder. And it can work for you in a similar way.

I started out using music to sooth me into slumber when I suffered from bouts of insomnia. These were evenings associated with high tension or stress produced anxiety. To deal with that problem, I bought an IPOD Touch which set me back around $150. I permitted myself the luxury of one album download each and every month. I built a nice library as me passed. Simply pull out your IPOD, pick an album, set it to low volume, and doze.

It happened every me that my muscles, rather like a clenched fist, started to relax. My state of mind, delirious racing thoughts, delusional fixations, or auditory hallucinations, started to decrease after only fifteen minutes. Further along, I began to breathe more deeply, I covered myself in a blanket, switched off the IPOD, and went into a slumber.

Experiment with different sources of music. Particularly useful are CDs of earth song. These might include one recording the sounds of the ocean, another entitled "Mountain Stream", or "Tropical Rain Forest". Put these CDs on something like a Phillips Entertainment Center ($100) which will automatically turn itself off at the end of the CD. Practice deep diaphragmatic breathing while you allow your imagination to people the night with the creatures making sounds in the background. Keep it a soothing low volume. You will discover how powerful earth song can be in controlling agitation, the depressions of a bipolar syndrome slough, or intense manic thought pa erns.

Another source of music might be your laptop or personal computer. Such websites as ITunes feature free streaming radio stations. For an interesting effect, try tuning in to some alternative music, something like John Di Libereto's "Echos" radio show on National Public Radio. The fascinating sounds and rhythms you hear will distract you from your current fixation or delusion, permitting your psyche to relax. Space music is particularly good for expanding the soul and relaxing those pent up emotions.

Almost daily, I find myself taking a calming walk with the IPOD on scenic trails and walkways near my home. Explore your area for natural beauty and scenic locations. As you listen and walk, you are garnering the benefit of music and exercise in centering your psyche, flexing your emotions into a semblance of contentment, deriving some muscle relaxation naturally resulting from usage. See for yourself the benefit of a daily musical interlude. Do not hesitate to use music in the car, while shopping, or when sitting in your comfortable recliner.

I found from experience that classical music, particularly harmonic and traditional compositions, were best for engaging me when I was troubled or thrashing it out with some symptoms. You cannot pay attention to auditory hallucinations and Beethoven's Spring Symphony at the same me! So I began to learn about different composers, choosing the ones I liked the most. I love Mozart, Sa e, Strauss, Haydn, Bach, and a host of others.

In fact, along with this new hobby, I began a ending free live classical music concerts offered by a nearby music school on Wednesday afternoons. I brought along a brown bag lunch. I met many new acquaintances at these events.

Gradually, my need for music as therapy increased. I began to learn piano. I bought myself an electronic piano for the home. The local senior citizen organization, Oasis, provided inexpensive courses in piano by a wonderful lively music teacher. I progressed to playing simple tunes to myself with headphones several times a week. At this writing, I have completed 30 lessons and am practicing Peter Tchaikovsky's "March Slav" and the popular folk tune "She Wore a Yellow Ribbon". Extremely proud of myself, I look forward to continuing to learn.

But my recovery took an even bolder step pursuing a new love for music in—joining my local church choir. That's right! I had been an alto as a young girl in high school, enjoying choral singing as a required course. Now I have auditioned and been accepted by a group called "The Contemporary Choir". We practice for two hours on Monday evenings. We perform usually once or twice every weekend. It's a wonderful congenial bunch of talented people. We are very friendly and rapidly becoming friends. This makes for a feeling of accomplishment or competence along with that marvelous feeling when singing in unison for the appreciation of the public.

You too might find a gradual development of mental health with bringing music more into your daily life. Music is a potent weapon. It can banish psychological proclivities and give you much relief from your symptoms. Start as a passive listener and see where the music takes you.

One word of caution–you may discover, as I did, that certain modern classical music, dissonant and upsetting, increases symptom flare ups. You might also notice that bebop, rap music, or offensive lyrics make you most irritated and "churned up". Trust your instincts and avoid any music which is highly repetitive, for example, Phillip Glass's compositions. Listen only to what makes you feel good.

Good luck exploring! I couldn't live without daily music–more and more!

The Joys of Gum (2014-09-28 15:06)

I long wondered why athletes in baseball, football and other sports habitually chew gum. Now I know! I am a habitual gum chewer. In a week's me, I go through almost $4 worth of the little wads. It's an expense I consider to be for therapy.

When I started, I was working a 9-5 job as a word processor in a little cubicle. The job required fierce concentration and speed. Once I started with my Trident, I found myself working long periods with ease. As soon as one piece grew stale, I replaced it with another. Sugarless, it didn't really put any weight on me. I knew my teeth were safe from decay germs.

Chewing gum is good for relieving stress, tension and anxiety. A good pal, it's easily carried in a pocket, purse or glove compartment. When you chew, your facial muscles are first clenched then released. It helps the relaxation reflex.

It is well known that mentally ill people are smokers at a higher percentage than the general population of the United States. The cigarettes relieve boredom, help stop anxiety or panic, and give something to focus on other than your alarming moods or delusional thoughts. But, as is evident, smoking is bad for you. It destroys your health over me. Someone who smokes a pack a day is going to wind up in the morgue sooner than others.

As mentioned in former posts, my belief is that smokers have a latent, subconscious desire to harm themselves. They are knowingly hi ng their lungs. It's sheer masochism.

In operant behavioral conditioning, a technique employed in the clinical laboratory, one signal (like the urge to smoke) is followed by a new response (grabbing an electric cigarette) rather than the prior one (smoking a tobacco cigarette), followed by a reward–possibly a piece of candy. Over me, the new habit replaces the old. And so too, the urge to smoke, which is based on a chemical dependency on nicotine, lessens.

I suggest you listen to your better self (or that little angel sitting on your right shoulder!) as well as your loved ones. Kick the habit with help. Talk to your regular doctor. Ask for a prescription for the nicotine patch or nicotine gum, which is often 100 % paid for by your health insurance.

Get into chewing gum instead. You will find that it serves you well in the future. You will feel better, look better, and live longer.

The Effect of Security on Schizo-Affective Hallucination (2014-12-09 11:06)

I recently landed a long-term temporary assignment at my job. My chosen profession is being a teacher. Much to my surprise, the incidence of auditory hallucinations per day quickly dwindled to next to nothing.

As a "toolbox" strategy, I self-check myself daily, recording moments of hallucination along with emotional flux on a time line. At each entry, I rate my "psychotic" state on an index from 1 to 10. Ten indicates I am full-blown psychotic,

while 0 indicates that I am totally at peace, psyche-wise.

Much surprised, I noted that each day was coming in on average with a P Zero rating. In this way, I discovered that what drives or fuels my schizo-affective disorder is the stress and instability my job brings–when I'm hanging helplessly between assignments, not knowing what tomorrow brings.

In contract, when I am certain of the next week's schedule, with a committed employer, at a post I can fulfill easily to the best of my abilities, my spirit soars, I am "in my element" and my disorder recedes to the background or simply disappears.

In this way I became aware that there are environmental triggers making my mental illness. Additionally, I realized that this had been going on for a long me. In reviewing my unstable, homeless past with rejection by cherished family members and social isolation–I understood that my life experience had made me sick. To be more precise, I had dormant, latent susceptibility to schizophrenia and my life had triggered the whole thing.

This is not to say that I now am "cured". But, for certain, I prefer to live a humdrum, routine, predictable lifestyle so as to avoid the painful daily confrontations with weird voices I am used to. In some sense, like an autistic person, I thrive in a predictable universe. This, along with the solid assurance of daily income earned–leads me to my "P Zero" place.

You, too, can discover key elements leading to your better recovery from mental illness.

Oversleeping Eliminates Auditory Hallucinations (2015-06-02 19:02)

For the past six months, I have averaged over 10 hours of sleep a night. Actually, it's closer to 12 hours. There has been a marked improvement in my mindset, focus and clarity have increased and the incursion of vague, distant or close auditory hallucinations has just about vanished. Try oversleeping and see if it changes things for you! I utilize a small dosage of Melatonin to hormonally induce sleep.

Actually, it's a bit of a sacrifice to give up that big a chunk of me for non-activity but the pay off in mental health more than makes up for it.

Oh, the Joys of Silence! (2015-07-06 17:28)

One of the most profound "balms in Gilead" is silence. As personal history dictates, tons of it are necessary for a cure to mental illness.

In keeping with that idea, which historically dates back to the me of the shepherd boy David and crazy King Saul of the Israelites–

Perhaps the sweetest place to live for a mentally ill person would be a sole owner residence surrounded by a lot of empty land.

Now, it's a proven fact that some people are hyper-sensitive to radio waves or emissions from light sockets, electronic devices or cell phones. They suffer a great deal when near electric wires or computers. Some choose to live in special communities nationwide where technology is voluntarily banned or restricted.

Strangely enough, this ailment parallels the sensitivity of some of the mentally ill, particularly those prone to auditory hallucinations. I speak from personal experience. Being in a woods, or on a remote beach puts me in heaven because those voice subside.

White noise, or the output of a neighbor's television can become enmeshed in the imagination of a mentally ill person and cause ruckus.

The ideal solution would be to purchase a remote cabin, an idyllic little cottage by the sea shore–or a deserted island. In days, weeks or months the symptoms will subside.

God bless silence! Not to suggest that the mentally ill person purposely make him or herself deaf. You see, the vibrations of sound s will travel in through bone conduction. The skull reverberates.

Along with relative silence, resorting to soothing harmonic music will modulate emotional symptoms and sine curves.

Experiment with silence on your own. At times, late at night, with a slight flare up of hallucinations, I dig out my wax ear plugs, put them on, and withdraw quickly into self-focused and centered restful sleep.

Experiment–that's the key word. Cure yourself, my dears!

The Calendar (2015-07-07 16:04)

Here's something you might try to structure your life. My day revolves around a cheap notebook of lined paper. It's my calendar book.

You know, mentally ill people tend to float into the ozone if there's nothing specifically happening at any given time. They indulge in fantasies, embroideries, then delusions which affects their mood–and waste a lot of thought and feeling on phantasms.

How nice it is to structure your me–your day. It gives you a new purpose, you find constructive and positive things to accomplish, and you–have a life! (A good lifestyle, a well-planned rhythm to your day).

My calendar book has about two days on each page, handwritten in. For example, "Saturday–7/7/15). Then I plan out the month. I put in my benefit payment, my payroll days, my doctor appointments, and the days I'm going to be away traveling. Each day has about fifteen slots for times. I put hours next to the activities.

But wait just a minute! This calendar can evolve into an even more useful helper. You can put in reminders to pay bills, to make phone calls to someone, or to do chores.

After a while, your week is pretty full and–ta-ta! You have a life!

I recommend you try this soon. There are calendars which come free with Windows for computers. I use this tool to sketch in things I have to do, or what's happening months in advance. When do I plan to wash the rug? When can I think about returning to my Orthopedic doctor for a new round of injections? When can I get dentures. Great stuff like that!

There's one more use for the calendar. You can record days you had a hard time, or fears you are having, or something you imagined or heard. No one will ever judge you for this record and, like a journal, it'll remind you of why you need to structure your time in the first place.

If you structure your time daily, the calendar will give you a plan for the day–and I think you will see a gradual decrease in mood swings, delusions or hallucinations. Your head will be on straight, you'll feel solid about yourself–and you will function in a more normal way. When people perceive how well organized you have become, they'll tend to forget you have a mental disorder. You won't be acting like an invalid or vegetable.

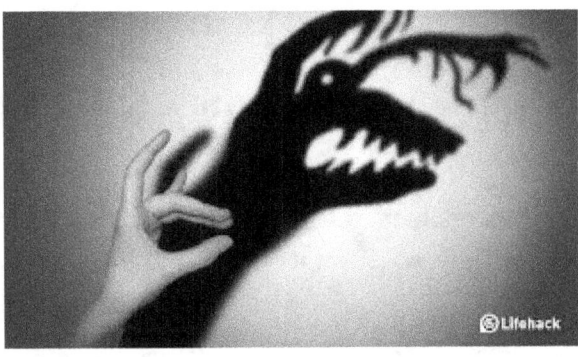

Chapter 19: SELF IMAGE

Continuation of the Subject of Yoga for a Mental Patient (2014-09-11 20:56)

A bit of humor in "mental patient" as a designation. No one should be called that, but there's a big stigma for those with a mental illness in our modern day society.

Why would you of all people want to do yoga? Well, consider it to be something like having a "tune up" for a car. It "degausses" the brain, resetting it to a new equilibrium. This is accomplished through practicing the hatha yoga postures regularly. But beware, be wary–there are a lot of phony yoga centers on the horizon. You should avoid Bikram yoga,

where work outs are provided in a hot house temperature heated room. It will make your mood rather extreme. It will not be good for your state of mind if you have a mental illness. Much better would be the choice of integral yoga, traditional yoga, or westernized yoga. If you want to see how you feel, take a class at the local YMCA, or buy a DVD and try a bit of it on your own. UTUBE has many excellent yoga videos for free–and some can be done in a chair sitting in front of your PC.

You will notice that your sensory perception is enhanced. You will feel calmer. The breathing tempo will be slow and regular by the me you finish an hour's class. There will be carry over of this good feeling you now have for several hours–maybe the rest of the day. You'll feel a whole lot better, your mood will have improved and you may find that you've "broken through" a delusional thought cycle.

Chapter 20: RELIGION

The Dangers of Spiritual Practice of All Faiths (2014-09-15 14:30)

Some of the spiritual practices discussed here include fasting, meditation, mindfulness, doing good works, giving back to the community, prayer, self-mortification, ascetic life style, keeping silent, and living a monas c life.

I recently started self-checking, as I am in recovery from a Schizo-Affective disorder which is mild. Since I am not taking medication every day and no longer seeing my psychiatrist, I must keep tabs daily on my condition. I use a simple 1-10 scale to gauge the level of psychosis. I am proud to say that most days are at a 2 level. This translates for me into meaning that occasionally, there are some auditory hallucinations.

However, without medication for a week or more, my brain simply begins to dysfunction and produces an intense delusional monologue coordinated with huge auditory hallucinations. These just pour in and incapacitate me to a large degree. Some of the symptoms which indicate that I am getting into a dangerous state of mind are a tendency to intensely pray, stop ea ng, or fixate on religious objects.

It is certainly a sign in many schizophrenics when they have a megalomania based on their identity as gods, angels or "spiritual beings".

In my youth, when the schizophrenia was just beginning to manifest, I devoted myself to the reading of religious books from the "Eastern Occult Arts", believing my psychosis was evidence of an "ESP ability" which I wanted to possess. I then became a strict vegetarian, gave up wearing leather, began to practice yoga, and denounced my Jewish background.

In spiritual practice of many faiths, there is prayer, fasting, a regimented ascetic life style, and devotion to a daily schedule which may begin as early as 4 a.m. and last well into the night. From experience, I can assure you that several facets of this lifestyle will negatively impact on your psyche, increasing schizophrenic symptoms. Loss of sleep has negative impact on you. Fasting will increase the intensity of your feelings and mood, with suffering and deprivation from comforts. Repetitive prayer such as Japa or reciting a mantra will turn the mentally ill person into a zombie.

For the schizophrenic, the "middle path" is wisest. Be kind to yourself and your psyche will be kind to you. Eat 2 or 3 small meals daily. Sleep at least 10 hours and take naps if you need to. Pray for short half hour spurts. Don't fixate intently on any object, idol or mandala. The middle path will compensate for your psychological weaknesses.

The monas c life is not something a mentally ill person may pursue with any hope of success. Rather, find a secular lifestyle where you can give back to the community as a volunteer. Use your God-given talents to teach, aid, fund raise, or serve. You will feel satisfied and closer to the Lord.

Perceptual Changes Resulting From Spiritual Practices (2014-09-19 00:21)

Continuing in the vein of exploring changes to you brought on by meditating, doing hatha yoga, practicing mindfulness through Zen walk, and more–well, there is actually a great deal of change in perception brought on by these. Some good, some bad.

Let's explore the good first. I would hazard a guess that you are not particularly "spiritual". Well, maybe you should be! I think many turn to God in some manner to find a cure for their mental illness. In desperation, they latch on to the common faith imbued in our Western culture. Or perhaps they turn toward the spiritual practices of Asia. In either case, fas ng never truly hurt anyone–as long as it's not bulimia where you are eating and then making yourself regurgitate because you have a twisted body image and think you must be extremely thin. Fasting is a form of purgation–and if you do it sensibly as taught by the three major faiths: Christianity, Judaism or Islam, you may find you are more regular for one thing, and perhaps something more. You might find your perceptions are refined–as if they've been given a good scrub. You'll see better, hear better and sense things tactilely better. Along with that, your smell sense may be keener. Indeed, after you have stopped fasting and eaten lightly, you might feel rather energized. Your balance may also be much improved. You may lose headachy irritable feelings. All from a modest fast!

Good accompanying meditation might include better concentration, memory and ability to think abstractly. You will notice that me has slowed down. Enjoying long moments afterward, you may dive into the depths of a profound serenity or contentment. This may lead on to a contemplation of nature which makes you feel real pleasure. Meditation also makes you feel refreshed. You may not need to sleep as much as before. But, perhaps, you may choose to sleep more because it is more tranquil, more free of lurid vivid nightmares or dreams. Your tension or stress level have gone way down into the normal range. The more regularly you meditate, the longer the effect will last. Your whole personality may se le into a quiet capable range of thinking with fewer delusions or emotional explosions.

Good accompanying hatha yoga practice on a regular basis is having a stretched, toned and supple body to live in. Your consciousness will center on your breathing. Your controlled breathing will lead to better intake of oxygen. Your cells will be awash with "Prana", the energy of the universe. By gaining control in poses and postures of your body, you will indirectly establish control over your psyche. This may balance a bipolar person. It may also eliminate some extreme mood swings, behaviors and delusional thinking.

What is bad about the above practices? Well–if you do too much, your body will rebel. Your psyche will harden into a stubborn ball of psychological difficulty. It may be too much to demand from yourself. It could cause to become delusional and feel you have an ESP ability.

Perhaps you will imagine you have a direct connection with the Lord—and auditory or visual hallucinations may result from meditating too frequently or too long.

At best, you might ask a friend or family member to monitor you weekly to see that you are "on an even keel". As mentioned in a previous post, all the good results mentioned above will be yours if you practice moderation. The middle path (discovered by Lord Buddha) leads to just as much insight and improvement as the modern human being can hope for.

Yes, I believe spiritual practice is good for everyone. It is one of the doors which lead to a cure. A cure is possible over me if you build a "toolbox" of techniques, habits, practices and activities which counteract the results of the chemical imbalance in your brain–the root of mental illness.

Remember: sometimes the brain becomes unbalanced because we have a history which includes certain traumatic or twisting episodes which hurt us extremely or injured our psyche to the point that the suffering became a chronic condition. With talk therapy, psychological analysis of the past may produce a catharsis which results in your brain achieving a new plateau of balance chemically. This will be explored in future posts.

But for now, why not give yourself an experience by trying a fast for a day? Simply refrain from solid food and treat yourself to juice smoothies made with raw fruits and vegetables for one day. See how you feel after you break your fast with a nice light meal at sundown.

Also, find a yoga class nearby to try it out. Maybe it will be free–or cost $10 or more to come once as a guest. Don't be shy–or go with a friend. Wear comfortable loose clothing like you wear for gym, kick off your shoes, borrow a yoga mat and try your best to do the poses. Afterward, check yourself and see the subtle changes the class has caused. I think you will be pleased with the way you now feel.

If you want to learn to meditate, there are many good books about it.

And there you go–you are on your way to becoming a scientist! You will be exploring ways to recover from mental illness in the future, using yourself as a guinea pig. Your doctor can't do all the work for you. Nor does he or she have all the answers! It's up to you to find the door, the gate, the path to wellness.

More Spiritual Practices To Modify (2014-09-20 18:56)

The Catholic has his rosary; the Hindu, his japa beads; the Greek Orthodox, his worry stones. The form of prayer which is prolonged, repetitive and frequent is a must to avoid–that is, if you are a mentally ill person. The effect will be apparent after a while. It will take the form of enhanced psychosis. You may have auditory, visual or synergistic (all senses) hallucinations.

Of course, you'll exclaim "I've come close to God! I'm having a religious experience–an epiphany!" Well, please be aware that in the realm of higher consciousness there is an element that spiritual adepts call "maya" or illusion. There is a possibility that you will "achieve self-realization" or experience "Samadhi" or reach the plane of higher beings. It will be harder to distinguish a genuine religious experience from a delusion. Only by speaking to your spiritual mentor, a cleric, a guru, an imam, can you hope to ascertain where your psyche is at.

Another spiritual practice which can produce exaggerated psychotic symptoms is the vigil. Whether at a late Mass during Holy days or done with a group, the key feature in this practice is a long period of relative idleness or boredom. It might be combined with a fast, candle lighting, religious services or rites, or inactivity while sitting or on your knees. These produce in the mentally ill person a tendency to fixate, go into a trance-like state, or experience long delusional sequences of thought which may or may not have something to do with God. It's best you avoid such messes.

There is nothing wrong with praying to God. Nor is there anything wrong in sitting in front of an altar for an hour.

You will bring it off successfully. Simply avoid going to extremes and your symptoms will be that much more reduced! Take it from one who has experienced and experimented for over 20 years.

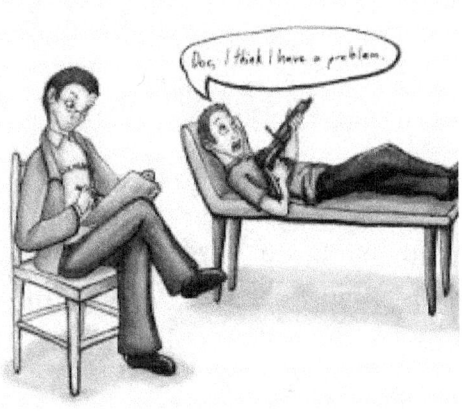

Chapter 21: LIFESTYLE

Some of the Watering Holes (2014-09-17 00:19)

A person who is mentally ill often finds the stigma unbearable. On top of that, the lack of friends is endemic to the condition. Also, family members may abandon or shun their needy, dependent and sick relative. For the person is just too hard to deal with, conflicts may be chronic, inexplicable behaviors infuriating, and actions leading to arrest or complaint problematic. Thus, the "m.i." (mentally ill) person winds up alone.

Now it needs to be said once—that the dependency is part of the illness—something which must be unlearned. Becoming self-sufficient is mandatory to resuming the semblance of a normal life. Parents may be crutches heartily tired of that role. It is understandable why so many negative emotions attach to the mentally ill. consumer.

Some of the places where the mentally ill consumer might find relief and growth include group therapy sessions, agencies built to offer classes, services and counseling to the mentally ill individual. In Rochester, that is the Creative Wellness Opportunities Center, an offshoot of the Mental Health Association. There are many others too numerous to name. Additionally, there are adult education classes offered free, internet chat rooms and post boards, and coffee houses where one can have a cup of coffee and some good conversa on with a stranger. Libraries are fine places to explore. They offer free lectures, film screenings, discussion groups and club meetings for free.

The greatest need in the desert of mental illness is an oasis; a watering hole. I have mentioned several above. It takes a certain amount of "gumption" to venture forth and explore possible places to visit. Many mentally ill people cannot bring themselves to get out of bed due to depression. What you need to do is start with short walks with the dog, chats with a neighbor, answering the phone, and the like.

I would recommend that, for starters, you try visiting a self-help support group. In this meeting of peers, all whom have acknowledged they have an illness and problems galore, you gain a feeling of belonging.

Some of the things a mentally ill person needs to make progress and get well are: A feeling of belonging, a sense of worth, and a sense of competence.

At all the places mentioned above, you get the ample chance to belong, to have a better self-image, and to do things which when accomplished give you a feeling of pride.

I hope you will, if that mentally ill consumer is yourself, take up the task of stepping out and visiting a water hole soon. For, after all, Man (and Woman) cannot survive without water.

Avoiding Bad Water (2014-09-17 14:02)

Why are so many "mental patients" smokers? Well, it relieves the stress, reduces tension, and eases boredom. I think there is also a masochistic tendency in the mentally ill which encourages them to hurt themselves subconsciously. Don't blame yourself for your mental illness.! Try to use one of those new tobacco-less cigarettes if you must.

As mentioned elsewhere, one should seek out the water of social interactions through visiting counseling centers, day programs, and joining clubs. We must practice our retarded social skills to get well.

Now, regarding "bad water", I'd mean that to represent some of the means of self-medicating a person with a mental illness utilizes. Alcohol, in all its many shapes and forms, is not good for you. Particularly, if you are on medication, chemical interaction will produce a pronounced effect which may, in fact, kill you. If you have deliberately stopped medication to take a vacation without permission from your psychiatrist, you may find yourself reaching for a beer when symptoms such as anxiety manifest. Don't. Keep away from bars, please. And when at social occasions, stay clear of the champagne flutes or mixed drinks offered. Alcohol maximizes symptoms including hallucinations, extreme feelings and panic attacks. There is no good in drinking it.

All right. I should get off my "high horse". I am not a temperance lady from way back. But I have learned to lead a relatively "clean" lifestyle to reduce my symptoms. I just like being that way. Clear headed, without visual or auditory hallucinations, lacking delusional streams of thought. Way to go.

Food Considerations (2014-09-21 12:34)

What follows are some simple rules I have found useful in maintaining my stability despite the effects of a schizo-affective disorder with a bipolar component. Yes, food can have a tremendous impact on your mind, heart and body.

So many mentally ill people overeat. Some do it is out of boredom because they are unemployed, relatively inactive, and dealing with long periods of hospitalization in wards with limited options for exercise.

That aside, they often pick the wrong sorts of foods to eat. Pasta and starches, refined sugar goodies and ice cream, whipped cream desserts–all these put the pounds on. A mentally ill person should strive to stay   "mean and lean".

To do so, I recommend that you embark on "The Weight Watchers Program", offered online and at a nearby weight loss center. The positive impact of this program cannot be denied. Take me, for example. I have lost 21 pounds gradually, changing my eating habits and lifestyle to something much more enjoyable and positive. By eating a diet heavy on lean proteins, fruits and vegetables (or "power foods"), we can shed the fat and regain our former shapes–with a great new self-image. That alone is worth the modest cost per week to be a member. And you have that great weekly pep talk meeting with a Weight Watchers leader to encourage and teach you.

There are other paths. You could become a vegan for much less money. Explore that as well!

Besides that, there are certain foods you should avoid. Caffeine in all its forms can produce manic symptoms. Sometimes we crave that feeling. It is not good for a bipolar person. Seek decaffeinated soft drinks instead. Avoid regular coffee and tea. Instead, try light coffee and herbal tea.

Avoiding salt and high spice in foods can be calming. A rather bland diet produces a rather bland mindset. You shouldn't seek stimulation from the nutrients you are consuming!

And now a word about sugar. No doubt, you may find the need to consume a candy bar daily. Addiction to chocolate is, once again, an invite to caffeine to wreck havoc with your state of mind. Simply put, the rush of sugar in your bloodstream may produce manic symptoms and increased psychosis. Going off sugar will prove my point to you within days. Refrain, cut down, and switch to sugarless candies. Your body will thank you in the long run.

When we follow a healthful diet, we gain confidence in ourselves, maintain our best appearance, and move and function better in the world. It's worth making the change.

If you have arthritis you may find that the above diet program also eliminates a great deal of your pain. I was proud to discover, after losing the 21 pounds, that I no longer needed pain medication or wearing a steel and Velcro brace on my le leg. There was no more strain on the joint.

After all is done, you can treat yourself to a new attractive wardrobe. Taking pride in your appearance once more, get a haircut, a facial, a manicure—love yourself! It's part of getting well. Dress great and you will feel great.

Dying Through Social Isolation With A Mental Illness (2014-10-04 00:23)

I'm watching a documentary, Boomers, and it's a long series of in-depth interviews with personalities, all of which were born in the boomer years, 1947-1969. And as I watch, I'm filled, saturated in my soul by the input from an intelligent, charming, or creative mind speaking frankly in autobiographical fashion about his or her life.

The absence of such moments or conversations in my life looms as the biggest obstacle to any happiness. It seems ages have gone by since someone took an interest in me long enough to want to know my interior life, or to know what it is that makes me this unique person. That, in part, is due to the effect of my mental illness, my "history" (as they say in polite language), my pariah lifestyle.

Although I am in recovery, recuperating from many false dangerous notions which approached the aberrant, I cannot fully rejoin the human race because, let's face it, many doors are shut. In faces I see each day, there is no love, nor tenderness, or a hint of subjectivity. This is my portion. This was not my choice.

I know this now because I've just watched for an hour, drinking in, the offerings of deep wisdom, deeper insight and confidences from people anybody would be glad to speak to: Billy Joel, Erin Brockovich, Amy Tan, Maria Shriver and a host of others.

We touched tonight–I switched on. My psyche blossomed, bathed in the dew from these roses. But it was courtesy of the silver screen, only a documentary's blessing.

Tomorrow there will be nothing similar. There have been far too many days like that. My feeble attempts to get to know such people as my choir master at church have led to some angry, distancing gestures. No one really wants to be known, or to touch another soul. It's probably because we're all in our sixties or older, I tell myself.

And yet, I know that the insidious theme of mental illness takes away all the treasured moments, the intimacies, the feeling shares which so much ease and comfort the independent psyche. We so deeply need to feel ourselves as men and women of substance rather than the ghosts the illness's stigma makes us into.

Fight against the swaddling suffocation of loneliness. Fight to cherish and love your very self. Cling to your uniqueness and never lose courage. This is the war coming back from the edge of madness. This is the only option for the recovering loony.

Reflections on Job Suitability for the Mentally Ill Person (2014-10-06 18:53)

Sad to say, many mentally ill consumers in our society suffer from the effects of deep poverty. They are unable to work. Yet, work can be extremely therapeutic for them, restoring a feeling of competence and self-worth.

During the forty-five year course of my illness, I held scores of jobs. In my case, there was a problem in dealing with authority figures ("bosses"), based on a deep conflict with my father. However, I had a strong work ethic instilled from early childhood by the examples of my relatives. I therefore repeatedly got fired, resigned, and resumed the job search.

Nothing stopped me from accepting a position. Many of the jobs I held were menial, inferior to my standing as a member of the middle class. I worked to become independent of my parents. Above all else, I wanted to live on my own. This desire started at age 15. During the next ten years, I ran away from home several times. But that's another story.

Let's take a moment to review some general guidelines which might help you find work and keep a job. These are observations and opinions based on my personal work history. Also, it is based on the diagnosis of a schizo-affective disorder with a bipolar syndrome axis. Added to that is some social anxiety, oppositional defiance disorder (regarding a boss), and homelessness.

Yes, if you can work in a factory, it's a concrete form of repetitive work. You may enjoy the monotony. There will be few challenges or growth moves you can make from your position. The structured work environment may include a uniform, cutting down your need to own a wardrobe. There will be expected lunches and short breaks during the day. You will have no overtime and weekends free. Your paycheck will be delivered right on time, every time. This type of monotony or dullness may work in your favor. It will relax you, sustain you and give you a feeling of accomplishment each week. There is an opportunity to make friends with your blue collar associates. People are real, centered in the bare necessities of making a living. You might grow to appreciate such people. If you need to stimulate yourself, bring a book to work for those breaks.

A source of frustration for you might be working in the fast food industry. The job is high stress, at a rapid pace. Your disorder or problem may cause you to lack the ability to focus or concentrate on multiple step tasks in rapid succession. At the counter you will have to think on your feet and work a cash register—often a computer in disguise with many command codes to memorize. I strongly recommend you stay away from this group of jobs. You will be frustrated, unhappy, and stressed out. You well may fail.

Regarding working in the office environment, there's a lot of stability to be found as a word processor working in a cubicle. If you're suffering from social anxiety, then you may avoid it here. Also, this work is often repetitive and simple. Once you learn to copy something, you're well on your way. Paychecks are regular, the environment is carefully structured and regulated. You may have your break times and lunch hours to socialize with others. Limiting time alone with others will lessen your anxiety and help you succeed in making friends.

So too, in a similar vein, are jobs as customer service representatives at telephone hubs. Once again, you are in a cubicle with a computer, facing a screen. You deal with the public using scripts, reading off figures from the proper menu. You may well excel at this. The pace is steady, the problems easy to troubleshoot. Once again, work is well structured, with systematic breaks, lunch periods and schedules. You well may enjoy the distancing the telephone provides in communicating with others. No one is going to witness your panic attacks or minutes of phobia or hallucination.

In any case, there are hundreds of jobs which are potential success stories for the mentally ill person. Persistence, stubbornness, and exploration will lead to some position you can keep to make a living.

Working as a grocery store clerk is another possible entry level position which will lead you into the broad field of food service retail. You will enjoy working with food. If you are shy, you can work the night shift as an order clerk. During these times, much leeway in behavior, dress, and speech are accepted by the kind night manager intent on restocking shelves for the new day. You may even be able to occasionally help yourself to a free meal, at the boss's expense.

Retail stores are other places which provide a structured work environment. However, these jobs would require you to "spruce up" and maintain a careful poise interacting with the consumer public. However, as you are recovering from a mental illness, if you enjoy fashion or glamor, these jobs may give you great satisfaction.

Related fields–the beauty shop industry, the jobs of hairdresser, cosmetician, or perfume salesman are just some of the titles you might add to your resume. All you need to do is get some training in a trade school, get a diploma, and register for a license.

If you've ever watched the television sit-com "The Office", you might think working in an office could be something to do. Well, if you become an administrative assistant, executive secretary, or middle-level executive, you will need to be capable of multitasking and working under great pressure. Take it from one who has tried–these jobs are a tremendous challenge. You might do better as a mail clerk or word processor clerk.

Civil service jobs might work out for you. Take the civil service exams in your field of interest. Work for the postal service. Become a U.P.S. truck driver. These jobs come with free training, uniforms, and a tremendous feeling of self-respect. You might enjoy walking your mail route each day, delivering to people, exchanging hellos and gossip.

I hope I have provided some useful guidelines for you. For those of you who are already skilled professionals or "brains", this is what I would suggest. There is part time and flex-time. With part time work you might be able to refrain from work on days where you are displaying symptoms galore without penalty or loss of the job. Flex time is an arrangement with another worker, sharing the job schedule as you wish–two people holding one job at one time. Usually designed with the new parent in mind, flexible time is a fantastic way to earn income and lose job pressure.

If you keep standing up after you get knocked down, have a presentable appearance and resume, and continue to train yourself in job skills required, you will undoubtedly succeed at earning wages.

Later on, if you apply for SSD or SSI, the benefit amount you receive upon award of benefit will be based on your former work history. To gain a nice monthly benefit check, you will have to have had some sort of success in the past. For this reason too, I urge you to continue working although society regards you as a "misfit". Good luck, my friend.

You and Weapons (2014-10-21 14:50)

"Love and marriage go together like a horse and carriage," is the old adage, but "mentally ill and bearing arms" is an oxymoronic pairing. Yet, you as a consumer are susceptible to attacks like any other citizen. In fact, due to your penchant for poverty, homelessness and solitude, you may be moving in surroundings which are high crime areas. So comes a tome when you wish to protect yourself.

It is a right to life, liberty and the pursuit of happiness as dictated by the Declaration of

Independence. There is also a right to "bear arms, as in a militia" which appears in the Second Amendment. This has been loosely interpreted by the American Rifle Association among other groups to mean that every grown adult in the country has the right to bear firearms. Additionally, firearms may be used legally in self-defense without penalty of the law.

But, woe is me! I've got a M.I. history! There comes a me when you feel compelled to apply for a pistol permit. A heavy section of the application demands disclosure of any treatment for mental illness along with any related hospital stay or medical treatment. To lie on that document is a crime. The majority of mentally ill citizens can legally apply for a permit to carry a concealed weapon–but they will never be granted one. Like ex-cons with a rap sheet, they are in a section of the population forbidden to own a gun.

In the early morning of December 24, 2012, firefighters responding to a fire in West Webster, New York, a suburb of Rochester, were fired upon by 62-year-old William H. Spengler, who was believed to have deliberately set the fire. Two of the firefighters were killed. Mr. Spengler, an ex-con, had needed a weapon in the worst way. Through the tender ministrations of a girlfriend who applied for a permit and purchased several firearms thereby giving them to him, William was able to shoot and kill his sister as well as ambush others. Such machinations are commonplace where you have been blocked by a legal technicality. Perhaps this is a good thing in many cases.

But, buddy, there's of course–You! You're a nice refined person in recovery from a mild bipolar disorder. You were recently mugged in the hallway of your girlfriend's aunt's apartment house. You don't smoke, let alone do drugs. You'd like to travel abroad at night, or visit downtown in the wee hours of the morning to have a drink at a bar. What're you going to do? There's no way your application to own let alone carry a concealed weapon is going to be honored.

Well, my advice to you is–obey the law! Mentally ill people are not the most well-balanced emotionally. It is quite likely that you will go into a tantrum, a trance state, a delusional cycle, a manic episode–and seek to act out. I mean, it's much more likely by probability than the rest of the population. Some inopportune moment, carelessness, poor judgment–and you've committed a crime–then you are really in hot water!

It may be the case that you are a threat to others or yourself--at moments, rare moments. Having your finger on a trigger would be foolhardy. Let's compare statistics about all the perpetrators of mass killings at schools and theaters in the last decade. How many of them chose to end their own life shortly after acting out? More than half!

How do you live life like a declawed housecat? If you saw a mouse, you'd most likely run away and hide!

Surely every citizen has the right to protect himself! You can't expect a police officer to be at your shoulder when a crisis arrives. My advice to you is to protect yourself sensibly. Martial arts may be the door of opportunity where training gives you an edge. I myself took a Self-Defense Personal Protection Training course this past winter. Do at least that much. If you have greater need, proceed to earn a black belt in Judo or Karate.

Another source of self protection could be a large, smart, trained pet dog. No special permit to own one.

And, there is the "manly art of self defense" (boxing). Take lessons from a coach at the local gym.

Or, live with a sane friend, partner, or lover who is permitted to own and carry a handgun.

I heartily don't recommend archery or pellet guns. Though legal, they are not terribly practical. Bee-bee guns are inaccurate and would more likely infuriate an assailant. For the same reason, carrying a knife or bodkin, though legal, is unsafe in battle at close quarters, unless you are an expert.

Finally, pepper spray may be illegal in your state–it is in New York. Such things as "zappers" or tazers are usually legally restricted to law enforcement personnel.

Good luck! Grow your nails long for starters. Thank your stars that you are under some civic constraint. Things could otherwise backfire and ruin your life–or end it!

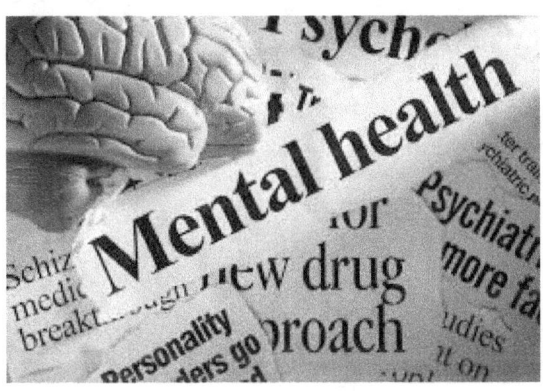

How Your Latent Schizophrenia Could Be Triggered (2014-12-10 13:56)

I want to take the risk of talking quite frankly about my past. There were certain choices I made as a teenager which affected my brain. These resulted in a dramatic change in my personality.

Researchers and scientists studying mental illness frequently write about the fact that there appears to be a dormancy or latency in a certain percentage of the population of the US which is a susceptibility to schizophrenia. The theory goes that if certain environmental triggers affect an individual, that person is catapulted by his or her own brain chemistry into a psychotic episode. This commonly occurs in the teen years or the early twenties of an individual's life.

In my life, the trigger for mental illness was drugs. I had a friendly next door neighbor who was a pot dealer. He turned me and my sister on to smoking marijuana when we were both around 16 years old. At the start, it was a nice way to become dreamy and gain a huge appetite. With the passage of me, exposure to stronger street drugs occurred. In my case, it was a new boyfriend who wanted to try LSD. I came along for the trip. He deliberately provided an overdose of the stuff. The result was that I tripped for about 3 days. Not only did I see fantastical colors and pa erns of dots in front of my eyes, I had extreme mood swings and scary perceptions, distorted by the drug. The boyfriend left me at home where I continued to have flashbacks for months to come. This was so destabilizing that my habits, my school work, my interests took a decided "hit" and at times I was barely able to function at all. Like that rock group, "The Beatles", I became interested in the transcendental experiences resulting from practicing meditation and yoga. I adopted a far eastern, mystical philosophy about life. I became so preoccupied with the reason for being that little else mattered. Dropping out of a community college where I had been making Dean's List every semester with an "A" average was the first effect. When I began to adopt a lifestyle of extreme asceticism, my parent's were mystified, completely in the dark concerning the changes they were perceiving. Baffled, they encountered a moody, argumentative, rebellious and secretive child. I then moved out of the house.

Some time later, although drug free, I had a full blown psychotic episode while living in a yoga ashram. Rejecting the "guru" and seeking to re-enter regular secular society, I had severe depression and strong delusional thinking. I then had a breakdown, requiring hospitalization in a locked ward. Seventeen ECT therapy sessions removed the depression, along with a lot of my capacity to remember. Some of the results were permanent. I was never after that able to remember telephone numbers at will.

I attribute the emergence of my schizo-affective disorder to the use of LSD and other similar drugs. I believe now that they altered my brain chemistry. Something with the serotonin and dopamine receptors got messed up. It would require decades of searching through different medication to find an atypical one which would restore more normal functions.

We can live our lives obeying society's rules and guidelines for good living or we can "take a walk on the wild side", as the song lyric goes. I believe now that if I had never used drugs like mesacline, marijuana, LSD, psilocybin–I would never have become mentally ill.

It's too late now to wonder what I may have become if I had not loused myself up. All I can do now is to witness my experience to others like yourself.

DO NOT DO DRUGS!

The Positive Effect of a B12 Supplement (2015-05-27 11:06)

I recently had the pleasure to hear a lecture by "La Diva Dietician" aka Marty Davey, MS, RD, LDS. She mentioned that some medications which treat psychosis often "leach out" the body's B12 reserve, leading to some symptoms of deficiency including poor memory, fogginess, and lack of focus.

I have been taking Olanzapine, one of the more unusual anti-psychotic medications for at least six years. I often complained about the retardant effects of even my small 5 milligram dosage daily. I felt that my competency and ability to do higher level abstract thinking were impaired by it.

However, in 2014, after a trial subscription to Newneutron.com, an exercise for the mind gaming website, I proved sufficiently to myself that my basic above average reasoning abilities were intact. Still, I was annoyed by the side effect of Olanzapine to increase lack of short-term memory (particularly with actions, names and numbers), and create a feeling of numb haziness in my presence of mind.

Well, I started taking B12 about a month ago–500 mcg a day. Much to my surprise, my daily over the counter multivitamin was only providing 7 mcg daily! In a matter of days, my feeling of oppressive fogginess, forgetfulness and memory loss had markedly diminished. The problem was gone.

I am still hoping to stop taking Olanzapine in a trial withdrawal this summer. The reason is that there are gradual side effects such as tardive dyskinesia (involuntary muscle spasms near the mouth area). In the meantime, supplementing with B12 in a 500 mcg tablet daily does the job for me. I'm much happier.

Postscript: My therapist, LeAnn Nelson, CSW, informs me that her aging parents resort to B12 injections which produce similar effects, retarding aging in a dramatic way. This correlates to my own experience.

As for Marty Davey, she has a good book available for those pushing 50 where she discusses many dietary factors affecting aging—she's a bit of a myth buster too! Check her out at: www.LaDivaDietician.com. (I only wish I could afford a consultation for myself with her).

Forced Leisure is great! (2015-07-01 10:32)

After a year of forced leisure with an SSDI (Social Security Disability) award, I have noticed an improvement in my condition.

It bodes well with Bipolar I to have long periods of silence, to live a regular schedule, without clusters of high activity, to have periods of boring repetitive hobby like crochet or sewing, and to enjoy such quiet pursuits solitary as reading books or watching television.

In keeping with this, sleeping at least 12 hours daily reduces delusions and hallucinations gradually over a long period of time.

A Gym to Join (2015-07-07 16:15)

I'm a member of a local gym. This is one of the greatest tools in my tool kit of techniques to control my mental illness. It's not just the escape from my apartment a gym affords.

At times, when I'm worked up or edging into a delusional fugue state (which, I admit, happens very rarely these days)–I head to the gym. Some grunt work, or honest exertion–calms me, centers me and focuses me.

I walk the treadmill, bike on the stationary bike, or use the elliptical trainer. The usual workout is an hour or so. There's all sorts of heavy equipment for weight lifting like Nautilus-style machines. Once a week, I weight lift.

Now, to me, that forty pounds I'm "shleping" with my left arm is my mental illness. Maybe it's an imagined enemy. Maybe it's my parents. Maybe it's just a deep delusion. As I go through rounds of repeats, I overpower the enemy. I come out on the other side victorious.

That's my secret. Besides all that, I'm toning my body, tightening up my belly–there's a little benefit from even a light workout. Appetite improves. Sleep is easier. Maybe I won't need to take my Melatonin tonight!

You will see how you feel after a workout. You'll be clearer in the head, more focused, tired but free of what ailed you coming in. Your heart got a workout–it's much healthier in more ways than one.

The gym is a good friend to the mentally ill adult. Open the door to a brand new hobby. Buy some athletic togs. You were an artist in high school? Join the jocks! See–now, your self- image has changed for the better.

Besides all this, a gym is a great crossroads. You bridge to all sorts of people, "normal" with whom you can socialize casually. Even an economy gym treats you to a Subway hero once a month, or free towels, or water.

If you join the local YMCA, you'll have the added benefit of team leagues, sports like paddle ball, tennis or basketball–where you can socialize and mix with your average Joes or Janes. There are also many group yoga classes to relax you. Try a spinning class–cycling in tandem with others to some loud rock music under the direction of a skilled trainer. The YMCA will run you a membership cost of $45 a month. It's well worth it–its therapy! Very economical therapy! (There are sometimes charity scholarships there for such as us).

And if you belong to Excellus Blue Cross/Blue Shield or some other health insurance carriers, your membership at a Y might be all paid for already.

Here's one other notion–you're shunned and solitary because you're mentally ill. There's chunks of your day to fill with something–not just eating cookies in front of television watching soap operas. Get a life! Just go to the gym! See how great you feel when you come back home.

Honestly, the change in how you feel will be something to amaze you every time.

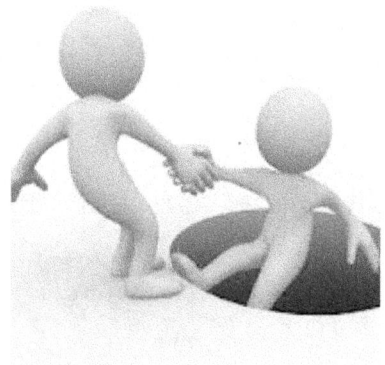

Chapter 22: RECOVERY

Re-entry, Recovery, Recuperation (2014-09-23 23:07)

If you have earnestly striven against mental illness, applying the techniques your therapist propounds, building an effective tool kit to modify behavior, lessen symptoms, increase a range of reactions–you may be told that you are now   "in recovery". Congratulations, but the work is just beginning!

You need to maintain your composure by employing all that you have learned. Perhaps you are no longer on medication, nor seeing a psychiatrist regularly. In my case, therapy was purely to check that I was self-monitoring.

This mental illness was an all-consuming antagonist in my life from age 20 to age 62. How hard I battled to keep sane! There were many milestones on my road to recovery. I took back my life brick by brick and erected a new dignity, a restored perspective. But you never really return to being the person who was first smitten. The human being coming through the tunnel of mental illness breaks through to the other side after an all-consuming battle–forever changed.

So how then will you re-enter the social milieu around you? How will you integrate into the lives of your fellow   so-called "normal" human beings? It isn't easy to contemplate. As is well known, the mentally ill lead lives of privation, isolation– stigmatized, labeled as being somehow on the fringe of society. They are greedy for a taste of the real life, desiring to share love with others, experience intimacy and friendship–prove their self-worth and competence in standing on life's stage and playing a role–any role.

I cannot provide all the answers here based on my own experience. In recovery for the next year, I am still struggling to stand with some modicum of privacy restored after decades. We will both try to find some answers in the posts I enter, categorize and save here.

The Bio-Rhythms of Recovery from Mental Illness (2014-09-26 17:07)

So, you've been re-evaluated and received a "clean bill of health" from the consulting psychiatrist. You did this to get a second opinion of your treatment plan. Perhaps that has been in place for years. The second opinion was fully covered by your health insurance. You simply phoned a local medical center and was referred to the appropriate professional to see.

Well, along with that your customary psychiatrist as concurred that your mental illness is now "in remission", your condition is best summarized as being a "light" one, and he feels that you can function well without seeing him. Besides, you were only seeing him to be monitored because you were taking medication.

Leading up to these developments, you had previously, with your regular psychiatrist's approval, weaned yourself off the medication you normally took, observing how it changed your functioning and managing your daily routine. You did manage to enjoy a nice vacation. Both doctors have agreed from the evidence that you can do well, even without medication, most of the me. So you are now virtually medication free although there is a pill bottle in the medicine cabinet, "just in case". Yes, you do occasionally take a dose.

But these relapses are rather rare. Now the talk therapist is only going to see you to monitor how well you are "self-checking". By this, I mean that you are judging your mental state constantly each day, watching that you don't get snagged by a delusion, develop insomnia, etc. The consul ng psychiatrist has given you a checklist of seven symptoms of trouble for a schizophrenic (or it could just as well be a warning sign list for someone who is Bipolar, or someone who has Obsessive-Compulsive Disorder and other conditions). You know what to look out for in yourself. Your talk therapist, a cordial friend by now, is going to see you for thirty minutes at two month intervals, then once at a three month interval, and then a last me.

After that, you'll have a phone number to call if you get into difficulty. There is also a "triage treatment plan" in your desk readily available to consult should you have a relapse.

You've managed to achieve independence. You have now reclaimed your privacy. It is wonderful to feel that you have worked out all of the kinks in your psyche. You can close the door to helpers almost all of them. What a great achievement after a long, arduous battle.

Just be sure to keep reading self-help books like Dr. Steven Hayes's "Get Out of Your Head and Into Your Life". Follow good health guidelines. Sleep a little extra. Read my other posts to strengthen your resolve.

And yes, my friend, let me wish you a warm "Congratulations"! You didn't attempt to do it until you felt you were ready. Fantastic!

About those biorhythms of recovery: You will not be climbing up a steep hill all of the time.

Sometimes you may fall into a slump or sine curve into some episodes of recurring symptoms. Slog it out–do not be afraid. The psyche has its own pace, its own tempo, its own means of healing. Things may come in waves, cycles, or simply steady progress. Be aware and don't give up on yourself, ever!

Sex in the City for the M.I. Person (2014-10-07 23:48)

The sexual identity of someone with a mental illness usually takes the form of either one of two extremes. Either they are conspicuously asexual, and have been without partners forever or they are aggressively sexual, working themselves into many casual relationships. Neither extreme is desirable or enjoyable.

We might speculate on the need for a man or woman to experience close intimacy. Many mental illnesses do not encourage that. A flaming schizophrenic is not easily engaged in conversa on, a preliminary step in forming even a friendship. The autistic man or woman frequently suffers from Asperger's Syndrome, lacking even rudimentary social skills. The bulimic person will not be attractive to others. Paranoids are never going to get close. Psychotics will be unreachable for long periods of time. Even neurotics have trouble building and maintaining relationships.

Yet, some people find an identity through sexual promiscuity. Many homosexuals prefer casual sex. Sex delays or limits pain, the inconvenient emotions of a delusional inner life. If one has a date, one feels important and needed. This illusion can pass as true love for a long stretch of me. Being desired may be preferred to being loved. One gets what one can in the "meat market" of the dating scene. But the mentally ill person rarely succeeds in keeping someone else happy. Stressing them out or providing chronic problems is much more likely.

The other end of the spectrum, living a dignified and aloof existence in solitude is, unfortunately, often the case for the mentally ill person. Well nourished, well groomed, but lacking the easy set of social skills required to flirt, perform as a lover and friend, or to encourage trust is a fairly accurate portrait.

The truth is, all human beings crave physical intimacy. Babies left alone in the crib untouched do not develop normally. Kids left with strangers cry for their nurturing parents. It's the type of attachment anxiety a mentally ill patient may feel toward parents and caregivers, even though he's in his forties. This is not a positive dependency on others. It replaces the give-and-take relationships "normal" people have.

In truth, with conscious effort, a person suffering a mental illness ("M.I.") can practice and learn the social skills which encourage others to approach, begin a dialogue, and maybe seek physical intimacy. With M.I., there will be a slower, more gradual passage in stages through the relationship until sexuality enters the picture.

I must say there is no easy solution to this problem. The M.I. person is frequently sexually deprived and frustrated. He or she may turn to masturbation as the only release of sexual tension.

This might lead into various prurient interests. The person with M.I. may become twisted, or turned into a voyeur.

At least, start by acknowledging the need. Second, work out your problems relating to others with a qualified talk therapist. Third, begin some social experiments through joining clubs, chat rooms, or dating web sites. Fourth–get your feet wet. Go on a blind date.

There is nothing simple about the hunt for sexual satiation, but it must be   attempted.

How Being Bi-Polar Can Rear It's Ugly Head Again (2014-10-13 14:01)

I have been through 2 bankruptcies and been forced through sheer hardship to pawn cherished jewelry items. I have also suffered homelessness through family disregard of my condition.

I went through a debt settlement company to deal with major creditors during the final process of bankruptcy. They insisted I take an online course in financial planning and living without credit. I passed. Since that me, almost 8 years ago, I have succeeded in avoiding the roller coaster ride.

Until now, that is. Yes, you'd think I'd have learned something from all that. But it seems that Bipolar Disorder, even in its mildest form, can come up and surprise the consumer in recovery.

Yes, during the summer I had need of a new used vehicle. A man made me an attractive offer I couldn't refuse. In signing the promissory note, I assumed that my present job would remain a source of valuable income each month. However, shortly after commencing the payment plan, it was obvious that all my spare money had completely dried up. I wasn't lucky enough to have money enough to buy groceries, let alone gas or postage!

Even though I could, on paper, afford the new car, I had been banking on my recovered condition. I was certain I'd be able to work at least three times each week. I'd make more than enough!

In fact, the job I held, per diem subbing, was extremely stressful and difficult, and my personality was not readjusting this Fall to the hardships or demands of my job. I was called onto the carpet in short order. A principal complained against me. I was forced to justify myself and my professional profile was denigrated.

So what did I do? First, I streamlined expenses. Then, I worked out new arrangements with my big creditors: a school where I took a summer course, the phone company. Finally, I put some items up for sale on Craig's List: a camera, a piano.

At this me of writing, I am surviving, dog paddling on the financial lake. I know I came very close to succumbing to my old habits. Still, I must be on guard each day now that I remember not to take a job for granted.

Bipolar Disorder Type 2 goes up and down like a roller coaster. In the past few days, I've been depressed. Knowing you have the tendency is enough to enable you to pull out of it. I spoke to my therapist by phone, and I'm good to go.

Just to close: There is no cure for Bipolar Disorder. Be very vigilant.

Failure of a Medication Vacation (2015-01-05 11:16)

There were 15 days off to my Christmas holiday break from teaching. I was eager to attempt to withdraw from my daily regimen of 5 mg of Olanzapine, for I had been very stable and consistent in behavior for days.

I lasted 5 days. When the frontal lobe thaws out and begins flailing its arms about, thrashing through old problems, worries and fixations–well, it is just too much to live with. I begin to see things in an extreme way. I take action. There are New Year's resolutions which are totally unrealistic–like giving up journaling. The habits in place give me structure.

A er resuming Olanzapine, what a relief! Gradually the extreme mood swings, the paranoia, the auditory hallucinations receded. It took a week before I was back to my old "mindless" self again. Yet, I am still intelligent. I simply don't have certain memories, feelings and thought patterns switch on.

On one level, I do not have at my disposal the creative spark, the intuitions, the deep musings which are the basis of my amateur writing career. At the same time, I do not have at my disposal the angst, anger, sorrow and lashing out characterizing my personal relationship with family . I do not write angry irrational letters or messages which get me into hot water.

I am resigned now to the regimen of 5 mg of Olanzapine daily. I am a bit of a wooden person on it. It is desirable to me to live a regular, normal, peaceful life.

As the experiment ends once more, I know that some pretty strange letters were written to my Bishop, and that I believed for a me that the monsters in my apartment house attacked me with radios and mentally to cause me to imagine that I heard all these weird messages. But then, that begins to fade.

Yes, perhaps I am a bit stupefied. I know I have no libido while medicated. But it is a blessing to escape the perceptual distortions and the unfinished emotional business which really has no solution in reality. I am a product of past history. With the medication, I can live a sane life on my own terms. And for now, that will have to be enough. I survive this way.

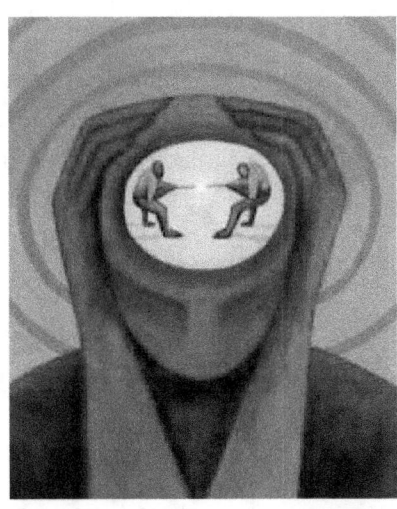

Re-Entry Into Society (2015-04-27 15:44)

When you have reached the point in recovery or management of the psyche where you are able to function for long periods on your own–with considerable tranquility or equanimity, balancing, coping, enjoying, sustained emotional stability–well–that's really something.

Still on medication after 4 months of relative self-autonomy, I can attest to the healing power of music and all the good work my therapists have done. I no longer try to be free of the Olanzapine. I do not doubt my mind is functioning admirably. I subscribed to "Newneutron.com", a website filled with games designed to flex the memory, the core knowledge, the executive function, the language abilities of your mind. I discovered that I was performing above average, with a steady rate of progress upwards. The only drawback of the medication was a pattern of slower than average reflexes. I had been self-deluded, believing that the psychiatric medication was making me a dumb wilted vegetable. Anything but! This last bit of nonsense cut me loose from continuing to progress down the road to total independence from the medical establishment.

I have decided never to have another companion, partner, husband or conjugal arrangement. I never want to lose what I have gained for myself and value my independence above all else.

But I have dated in recent weeks. I am seeking to resume some form of relationship which promises fulfillment in friendship and yes, possibly more.

The Brain – On a More Positive Note (2015-07-06 11:12)

In my previous post, I listed several causes of psychosis in the predisposed individual. The list was neither exhaustive nor complete. It is true that the excesses of youth can permanently damage the brain, disrupting the delicate balance of neurotransmitters, the stability of the hippocampus, or the perceptual apparatus of the mind.

I'd like to point to my own history to remark on the resiliency of the human brain.

And add a note of optimism. I have spent many years suffering from auditory hallucinations. I have had my core mind deeply disrupted, wracked by delusional material flowing in a steady stream for hours or even days. But–with patient plodding, careful adherence to a regimen of medication–the brain can and will bounce back. It has the capacity to recover it's balance, to "degause" and restore normalcy of function. It may take weeks, months, even years– but don't write off your own brain as injured or damaged. You may well recovery full use of your faculties in a clear, coherent mindset, balanced moods, realistic perceptions and executive function which enables you to become a successful human being.

Yes, the brain is remarkably resilient. The damage can and will be undone if you follow a medical solution to its optimum end.

A Disciplined Life Has Advantages (2015-07-08 10:10)

I live a pretty disciplined life. From the start, my life contained many disturbers and conflict-makers in the form of family members who contributed to my emotional and psychological development in detriment. It was a rather rocky ride. There were both verbal and physical abuses to a moderate extent on a regular basis.

My mental illness manifested when I was about twenty years old. I am now 64. It has accompanied me all my life. From 2007 forward, auditory hallucinations making havoc with my daily sense of self. Prior to that, a lot of "emotional grinding" in the form of negative personal events locked me into a pattern of grief, anger and frustration. But, with the help of much talk therapy, I worked through most of the feelings. With the right medication, Olanzapine, I toned down the sensory disorder.

And now, with the help of a disciplined lifestyle, I have reached a point of remission. The mental illness has, to a remarkable extent, let go of me. But I must live within certain set mental boundaries to make that happen. I have mentioned in other posts such things as keeping a journal or calendar, going to the gym–we must all construct a tool kit of methods to self-monitor and regulate our daily lives. Giving them structure is a desirable thing.

However, we don't want to live a life of rituals and routines like someone with a compulsory disorder. That would be going way too far.

And, I must add mention that I am not yet entirely free of auditory hallucinations. They're still there every day, just very far away and distant. They are significantly weakened.

But, living a disciplined life entails structuring your time to meet your dreams and goals. You must add clubs, hobbies and social activities which involve you with other people. Such internet websites as meetup.com are invaluable in your finding a group of people who share your interests whether it be biking, arts and crafts or handicrafts. Sometimes, people just like to meet to make friends. Yes, I realize it's not something you want to do. But–force yourself.

Regarding clubs, you can often find mention of these in your local newspaper or city website online. There are many clubs which meet at local libraries–so resorting to a library newsletter is essential to finding and joining a book reading club for the summer. Yeah, read the books!

All of this is good for you. Your psyche will respond to a regular routine. A large part of a disciplined life is waking up at a sensible morning hour. I find I am better symptom-wise when I arise mornings. I am essentially what I consider "normal". As mentioned elsewhere, I use a system of self-monitoring where I assign a "p value" to my state of mind. Usually mornings feature p zero. This wonderful free state lasts for several hours.

Having your three meals a day at routine times is good for your body. Controlling your weight by joining

Weight Watchers International may lead to a better disciplined eating pattern. You will slim down and have better nutrition. Taking vitamins regularly is beneficial. Not smoking will extend your life. Quit!

Regarding discipline, you may find that exercising once a day will help regulate your mood swings. Having to walk a pet twice a day might better structure your daily routine. Pets are good care givers too. Get a therapy dog!

All in all, I suggest you avoid those loose hours where you just sit and stare off into space. Find something to do, somewhere to go–for these moments are when you are prone to a flare up of symptoms. Or times when you are pensive, on a park bench, drifting off into memories of what happened with Aunt Sally, self-destructive or neurotic thoughts might possess you. You don't want to have that happen. So–keep busy. Not overly busy like an ant. Just enough scheduled and planned so that your day adds up to something, counts for something.

And with discipline, your self-control skills will kick in. I think you'll see a definite improvement in your state of mind. Mental illness is a form of self-indulgence. You give it permission to take over your soul. The mental illness will withdraw to its corner of the ring and stay there. Show it who's boss. YOU!

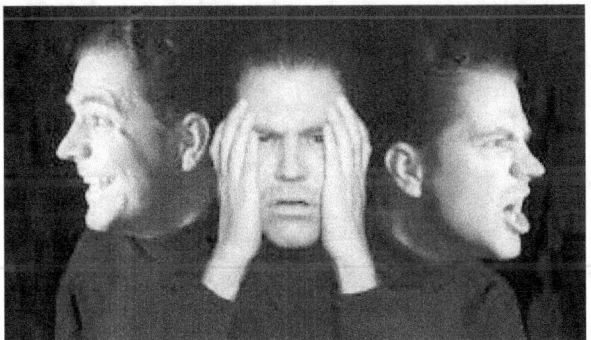

Chapter 23: SELF IMAGE

Self Hate as the Issue (2014-09-29 14:06)

Let's be frank about it! A person who suffers from a mental illness harbors feelings over me which are negative. I mean, besides the churning, roller-coaster rides of the bipolar mania and depression cycle, or the agitated anxious feelings of social anxiety. We harbor feelings related to our self-concept.

You ask yourself to be well. Your psyche refuses to comply. Despite your best efforts, a long time passes and you are unable to function, hold a job, get out of bed in the morning, relate to others. A host of problems face you daily. You cannot by an act of will force yourself to be in a new place free of hallucinations or delusions. So you screw up your face in the mirror, stop looking in that daily, and hate yourself.

You hate yourself in the many ways you describe yourself. I'm damaged. I'm an abnormal freak. I'm sick. I'm broken down. I'm doomed to be this way for the rest of my life. I don't want to live anymore being like this. This is the common flow of thought you might be sub-consciously thinking or feeling.

So you stop showering daily. You avoid brushing your teeth. You can't find the urge to shave or get haircuts. Your clothing becomes slovenly because you don't care to do the wash. You pick up the habit of smoking. You use cuss languages habitually as you are frustrated. In other words: you degenerate into a mess!

The appearance is directly a result of the negative self-talk. You need to change. I can't give you the universal key to make that happen. But I can show you that you need to make an effort. For hate is as damaging as sulfuric acid in diluted form. It will eat through your body and soul and leave nothing but a suicide attempt at the end.

Heap onto all this the reactions of others to your mentally ill condition. Your family may eventually get fed up and shun you. You may be divorced from a loving spouse who has suffered long and hard in forgiving and forge ng the many things you do when you are in the throes of it all. You may have been abandoned by family, children, and friends. This only drives the wedge deeper into your heart. You freely and consciously bear the social stigma of your illness. You are a pariah, an outcast–rather like the isolated lepers of Biblical times. You feel like someone has a bell and is ringing it to warn off any potential friends when you draw near.

I cannot tell you how to pull yourself out of it and love yourself. I can only tell you how I did it. For me it was a new found belief in Jesus Christ. I converted to Catholicism in my darkest hour as a homeless divorced derelict. You may find self-forgiveness and self-love in practicing your former faith or a new one.

I also suggest you pretend that you are in the army or navy. Self-discipline may take the form of sweeping the apartment once a week, doing the laundry in a group home, or shaving daily. Have some pride–do the simplest things for yourself. Reward yourself with a treat–a piece of candy. Believe it or not, you will get back on track.

The first step in getting well is loving yourself. Group therapy in the form of a self-help support group of peers will give you the life net you need to rebuild your self-image. You will make friends among the mentally ill. You will be accepted as a brother or sister. Do that for yourself too. At meetings, express your self-hate. Ventilate and get it out of your system. That will be healing for you. They will provide encouragement and the reasons why you must love yourself.

Finally, I will pray for the self-mutilator who cuts himself, the anorexic who starves herself, the depressive who crawls into bed for weeks at a time. You pray too. Prayer works.

Self-Hate II – "It's Not My Fault Because...." (2014-09-29 20:06)

We have already discussed some of the signs of self-hatred a mentally ill person may display.

To review: There are displays involving self-harm; derogatory remarks in response to social ostracism; many sorts of behaviors displaying a lack of basic hygiene; a deterioration of the physical appearance such as poor dress; a negligence in personal habits leading to alcoholism, use of drugs or cigarette addiction.

The poor self-image feeds on a spiraling cycle of thoughts and feelings, almost like a monologue which is intensified by the silence due to the lack of personal relationships or inclusions in social activities. These feelings may be raw, edgy with violent overtones, difficult to express, or impossible to deny. It might be that they seem to come from outside, or from a separate entity known only to you, or simply manifest as auditory hallucinations. It might feel like you have a new pal named Harvey the 6 foot pookah, an invisible bunny rabbit who followed Jimmy Stewart around in that famous movie from the 1940's, "It's a Wonderful Life".

"Why am I mentally ill?", "What did I do to deserve this?", "Why is this happening to me?" are questions demanding answers from your internal executive function or ego. You probably will read a great deal of published material on mental illness. Typically, a person like yourself in college might decide to become a psychology major. In an almost impossible quest to treat yourself, you might become enmeshed in the local chapter of the Bahai, or go to séances, believe in spirits, ghosts and esp. You'll consort with mediums, psychics, and all the flakes on the fringe of society. There may be a deleterious result to this. You might become filled with strange theories about your psyche, what is causing you to imagine things, hear things, or feel the roller coaster ride of the Bipolar disorder. You will increasingly feel the need for comfort. There is none to be found in drink, smokes, or intense physical exertion. You can't lose the problem in the gym–although it might be sidelined for a while. I think of the magnificent performance of Michael Phelps, the Olympic gold medal winner in Swimming in his struggle with Autism

Spectrum Disorder.

Finding solace in the arms of another will be another experiment. You will feel self-loathing as you run from unfulfilling encounter to encounter. You'll be stymied by what you say and do which offends, perplexes, disturbs or turns off your romantic partner. There'll be questioning about your sexual identity–and perhaps you'll find that you aren't highly sexed at all with very little need for physical intimacy. No, instead, you'll function like an android, a robot, a Vulcan– refusing to let yourself feel, loathing the times you sink into need or desire for another's company.

It's a bit like passing through adolescence–but much more rocky and intense. So you'll find reasons for self-hatred as the mental illness progresses. Schizophrenia often begins in adolescence. Not recognizing the signs or making excuses for what you have become lead to non-diagnosis until your condition is more extreme or advanced.

With involuntary hospitalization or confinement in jail, more sources for self-hatred crop up. You're a disgrace to your family, a problem, a failure, and a burden. How will you ever justify the pain and suffering you are putting your loved ones through?

How does this cycle of self-hatred end? Simply put, by loving yourself. You need to accept fully what you are capable of, confront the very real problem staring you in the face when you look into a mirror, and embrace the pain which comes with the mental illness.

This will take an extremely hard and long journey–the road to self-love, to recovery and reintegration into society on new terms. Maybe you'll not make it–maybe you will. If you love yourself, chances are you will avoid suicide, drug addiction, ac ng out or other myriad negative adjustments to mental illness–and you'll come out on the other side with something le to your soul–something valuable, something to be treasured and cherished–yourself.

Because, you know, God loves you. You are loveable. That's the god's honest truth.

Making a New Persona *a la* Bowie or Madonna.... (2015-07-06 17:40)

Sometimes the deepest roots of mental illness are found in your social environment. Quite likely, the dysfunctional relationships and intense conflicts with family members, spouses, friends or bosses have fragmented, damaged or destroyed parts of what might otherwise have been a healthy personality.

The mentally ill person is like a bombed building or swiss cheese in psyche. Sometimes therefore the healthiest thing that person can do is to create a new identity.

This person went so far as to a legal name change. She also changed her religion. Who cannot say newfound competence and wholeness have not been made in that major upheaval?

David Bowie, a renowned rock star, kept his fans amused for years in transforming himself and his appearance into various vivid personas like "Ziggy Stardust". It was a form of self-dramatization. He inhabited the personas at his rock concerts, wrote songs to fit their dreams, orientations and feelings, and lived vicariously through them.

Madonna, a world renowned pop artist, transformed herself into a single name persona with a sexy, sultry and "material girl" perspective on the world not in keeping with her personality formerly. It works to create a work of art which she transmutes into huge theatrical presentations. She is out of herself so to speak.

You may have to take such drastic steps as a name change or change of religion to produce a new viable life net for yourself. A life net is a group of positive supportive people in relationship to you who can enable you to better survive life's daily struggle. At the very least, you should extricate yourself from the dead or dying hulk of your personal life.

If you are in an institution, you may be under the control of family members. They may have power of attorney; you may be involuntarily confined. Your first step will thus be finding a stranger–an advocate or lawyer who specializes in helping such people as the mentally ill who have lost all their rights. And you do have rights. You need not be victimized indefinitely. (If you have been convicted of a crime, even so–there are court agencies and organizations to help you–though the battle for a new start will be more prolonged, difficult and troubled)

Make a project for yourself in recreating your own identity. It's a solid proposition on good footing with all the latest in psychological theory. You focus on a healthy new identity–in detail. Don't let your sickness control the thrust of it.

Dream a little, be positive–and find a way out of the wreckage of your life.

That's your job–your first priority in getting well!

Take this advice from someone who did just that–made herself well!

Chapter 24: COACHING TIPS

Schizo-Affective Flare Ups – Out of the Blue (2014-10-30 07:33)

Don't be disheartened. You awoke at 6 A.M., and a number of quick loud auditory hallucinations hit your groggy head. You knew you were properly medicated at the time, had slept more than enough hours as planned–and yet, here's a relapse in progress! What to do?

I do not have an easy answer for you. It's not totally brain chemistry. Lurking in your sub-conscious there may be some stressors struggling to become apparent. It's hard to know what's bothering you every moment in time. The relaxation of REM sleep, may release some tension in the form of a waking nightmare.

In my case, it was apprehension about an upcoming job assignment in one day. I immediately recalled how upset I had become almost two weeks ago when called on the rug by an immediate supervisor. I had thought the attack grossly unfair, and reacted appropriately–but it cost me some in balance. Ever since the episode, I had been kicking myself for fouling up on the job. This anger and hurt surfaced this morning in a wave of hallucinatory symptoms.

Like you, I carefully take medication and monitor my schizophrenic tendencies each day. Hey, if you aren't doing it–you're in recovery–you should! My method is very simple. On my desktop, I have a document called "threats". (It is called this because I perceive psychotic habits and events as an attack from the outside) While the day passes, if I have ANY symptoms at all–whether psychotic or emotional swings–I record them in a journal entry. Then comes the good part. I assign each episode a "P number". The "P" stands for "psychotic" and the number, which is 1 through 10, signifies how severe. Ten is a maximum psychotic event. Zero means I'm completely lucid, balanced and functional. I erase this document and start over each day. During the course of an average day, the number changes, ebbs and falls. There is no discernible pattern over the course of days. That's the nature of the beast!

One last thought: Don't beat yourself up about the lapse! The human brain is a very complicated organism. It goes through constant changes. If you haven't guessed by now–there is essentially no total cure for schizophrenia or schizoaffective disorder (a variant). I will probe more deeply into the nature of schizoaffective disorder in future posts. But for now–be kind to yourself. It happens. Know what to do when those times come. I go directly to my "threats" file.

After that, based on a reoccurrence, I begin to apply the methods of control carried around in my "tool kit". It may be taking a pill, or a soothing bath. I also try to trace the thing which is destabilizing me subconsciously. Sometimes successful. Sometimes not. Don't be hard on yourself. You are still in recovery.

Brain Chemistry (2014-11-14 09:40)

Yesterday, I had a rather trying time waiting on line at a government building. A check had been stopped after deposit in my checking account and I had no clue why. It meant $100 less a month–which was something I normally depended on.

Filled with adrenaline and cortisol, my brain went into overdrive and began working in a different but oh-so familiar way. Cortisol is the hormone which kicks in with stress. Adrenaline is the agent for increasing readiness to fight. It speeds up the heart and mind. Racing into a manic state, my mind began to manufacture a constantly changing series of imaginary scenarios to explain the attack on me. At least, it felt like that.

I began to experience something like a mescaline or LSD high. I must confess that while a teenager, *a la* Freud, I experimented with both drugs. Now, a symphony of auditory hallucinations began to play on me. I heard threatening words while on the waiting room line. I was warned that I was the target of a civil suit brought on by my ex-sister-in-flaw. In my mind's eye, many movies played out in gossamer ghostly fashion.

Familiar with this fugue state, I stolidly withstood the assault. I distracted myself as best I could with a magazine–a standard tool kit method. But it got to me! Fearful, I called a local lawyer and left her a message. Could I meet with her to discuss a pending civil suit? I was surely going to be a attacked by my enemies. After I hung up, I felt so foolish. (Wisely, the lawyer never phoned me back–she knew I had M.I.)

The crisis resolved into a comedy. At the customer service representative's desk, I broke into a smile. She informed me that they had put a stop on the check at my own suggestion in a previous visit. They had issued another and I would receive it the same day. I felt so foolish! I walked bemused to the car.

The chemical imbalance in my brain continued all day long. It was like a "trip". I counterbalanced it with tricks from my tool kit. I exercised hard at the gym. I took 15 mg of my antipsychotic medication—-3 times the usual daily dosage. I waited it out. Gradually, the hallucinations subsided. But I was in no shape to see people or work.

Nervously, I reviewed the warning signs of a schizophrenic relapse. These are:

1. problems with sleep–yep, I'd been oversleeping (12 hours a night); 2. Problems with appetite; 3. Depression-yep, 4. Problems with concentration, 5. Restlessness, 6. Tension or nervousness-yep, 7. Use of alcohol-a little in the past week, 8. Use of street drugs (like pot), 9. Hearing voices or seeing things that others can't hear or see–yep, very pronounced for 2 hours, 10. Less pleasure gained from things you enjoy, 11. Feeling people were watching you, against you, or talking about you–yep, very severe, 12. Preference for being alone-Yes, lately, 13. Arguments with others, 14. Inability to get your mind off one or more things

I had six out of 13 symptoms for about 12 hours. I decided not to pull the plug and phone in a medical emergency to my psychiatrist because it eased and went away.

But you can see what sort of horrible day I had. And you can relate, my friend, to that.

In closing, let me just mention my frustration with that swirling mess of chemicals in my brain. The imbalance of Serotonin and Dopamine. The influence of Cortisol. If only there were some method   to "degauss" the brain (like a television set with an electromagnet) or rebalance your neurotransmitters. These days, you can increase your medication and wait it out. That is all.

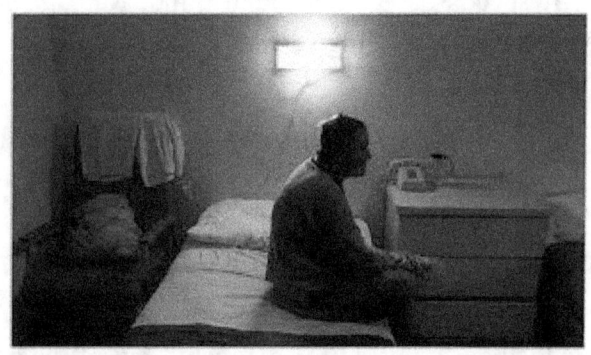

Tony Steel Helmet Lesson (2015-05-29 10:37)

For the past five years, I have struggled with a mild to moderate schizo-affective disorder with a bipolar axis. Significant challenges in my personal life led me to deal with both grief and depression. Social isolation has been part and parcel of my daily life.

To deal with my m.i., I developed a tool kit of methods which modify my psyche, diminish the symptoms and enable me to be happy. One of these for a very long time is an agency unique to Rochester, New York. It is called "211 Lifeline". If you dial that number in the city region, you will be channeled to a group of trained lay people for therapy and free advice. From 2009 until about 2012, I made scores of calls to 211 and I found stability return as a result of their unique personal touch, patience and dialogue.

One of the best therapists on the phone was someone calling himself Tony, an alias. No matter the number of times I spoke to him, he always retained his composure and patience with me. He treated me with respect, like an equal, like another human being.

As the months passed with using Tony, I commented upon his   "steel helmet" mentality. He laughed it off, but was pleased. Tony has his feet solidly on the ground. He is extremely practical, concrete and shrewd. Many a delusion fell by the wayside after he influenced me. Ultimately, I felt the desire to meet Tony in person. This, unfortunately, is impossible, considering the nature of 211 Lifeline. Tony remains to this day a mentor, role model and friend. He is a few digits on the phone away.

After months of tool kit care, my condition became milder and milder. I only called 211 Lifeline once a month. Not even. There was a therapeutic cure.

I have never met someone like Tony before, except perhaps for my father. His strong, centered and well-meshed personality, with clear opinions and judgments based on his own experience is what I envy. I would like to be less sensitive, neurotic and labile–I would like to have a steel helmet of my own to deal with daily pressures and tensions.

In the past six months, a new re-evaluation behind me, I see a therapist less often–just four times a year. I have a thick skin and a new helmet of my own, apparently. I just copy Tony. I remember his perspective on life and the world, and I borrow from his strength.

I hope you too find someone with a steel helmet to lean on.

Chapter 25: THERAPEUTIC THEORY AND PRACTICES

Against Freud's Theory of Sublimation (2015-07-01 10:27)

A Dismissal of Sigmund Freud's Sublimation
as a Source of Healing! It is invalid for a person to
pursue sublimation as a goal.

the person is beset by serious troubles or conflicts in his or her personal life, difficulties must be surmounted, solved and never ignored.

Someone took my kids away from me–and it was apparent murder or some crime of which I was a victim.

Those around me ignored the case and did not assist me in my endeavor to find my kids or keep them.

Rather than dealing with my ex-spouse and the criminals in my family, I pursued a college degree, throwing energies into becoming a better person, achieving a profession, and building a solid personality based on a religious conversion.

All well and good. From 1996 until 2011, I pursued this course of action. Due to it, I survived with some integrity, and new-found strength to live life.

However, the elementary conflict and crime were not resolved, and the anguish, long sub-conscious, re-emerges each day demanding a solution, justice or discovery.

And so, after reading and studying, indeed honoring Sigmund Freud his wise insights into the human psyche I must state unequivocally, from my personal example, that striving for sublimation, or seeking to rise above is not the primary goal or a road to satisfaction for a crime victim.

Only catharsis, whether it plays out in a violent act or some activity leading to resolution of the deep conflict one faces can be the valid pastime of an adult person.

Illegal "Psi" Research on Children (2015-07-01 10:29)

If you take malnourished children, afflict them, then stress them out, remove them from their parents producing attachment disorder;

Then place them into a hothouse environment of overstimulation, with enrichment, strong positive reinforcement, creation of new bonds of trust and loyalty with caretakers and surrogates;

If you administer drugs with pep up qualities, such as inhalers containing epinephrine for "asthma"; The result is that the kids kind of explode or implode and, like de-husked clams, become "open".

If this deliberate procedure is followed, you get little Shirley Temples, Judy Garlands and Buster Keatons, which, much like dwarf stars, burn very brightly indeed. In this state they can be manipulated through behavioral techniques like token systems to show "psi" or "ESP" qualities.

But really it is a retrogression to a more primitive *modus operandi* for the human brain, which becomes damaged;

It harms the child irrevocably. He is in bondage to his own five senses and displays proprioceptive disorders, and an inability to close the flood of stimuli, autistic symptoms, paranoia, psychosomatic illness and finally early "burn out".

Children are not batteries, and neither are they walruses. Such sins of technique are rampant and in-excusible, disguised as scientific inquiry or technique.

Recognition of these practices produces sadness in this writer.

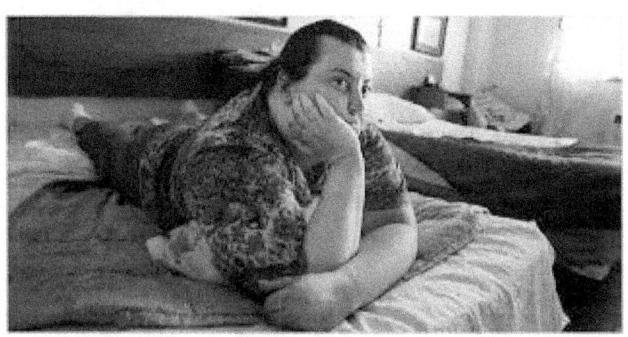

Construct a New Life Net (2015-07-01 10:33)

restructure
social   therapy:
my idea is:

that you can alleviate m.i. by restructuring the life net–actually manipulating the family system. You can add loving, doting nurturing mom, dad, sibs or friends–this will cure the patient.

In this new system, the therapist

1)   analyses the dysfunctional relationships and ends them;

2)   understands the dynamics between people;

3)   establishes a baseline for a healthy circle of supportive friends and families

4)   uses a database of volunteers, compatible people to insert into the patient's world;

5)   prepares and establishes the patient's trust and confidence in this new experiment;

6)   introduces the new partners in life;

7)   monitors and adjusts the life net

8)   observes and records progress periodically

All sans drugs!

My contention, the theme is:

In over 50 % of all cases of mental illness, a cure will be effected by restoring a quasi-

normal life net and lifestyle to the man or woman which lasts for years.

How to do this is the problem to work out.

There is no such therapeutic approach, I believe, on record yet.

Actually is.

Leary's early work in psychology expanded on the research of Harry Stack Sullivan and Karen Horney regarding the importance of interpersonal forces in mental health. Look into it!

Chapter 26: HISTORY

My History Summarized, "In a Nutshell" (2015-07-01 10:35)

It's been a long journey through a series of illnesses since I was about five. At first I blamed them on my mental illness. To this day I don't know whether suffering from afflictions including acute childhood asthma, hay fever, allergies, acne and scoliosis may have damaged my self-image. I only know that I was always considered "different".

In the age of "Flower Power", I too indulged in the types of so mind-altering substances which make you "cool". I relished "spiritual experiences", and subsisted on a vegetarian diet. Increasing impulsivity led me to self-medicate with bottles of brandy while a ending college. I wrote strange journals. I spent days without sleeping. My romantic life? Promiscuous sex.

It was all concealed from my parents. Even after treatment, they took no interest. There was no NAMI in the Sixties.

Living on my own led to a series of jobs, none of which I could keep for one reason or another. For example, the president of a menu design company caught me at my typist's desk reading the newspaper and canned me. I knew something was wrong with me but couldn't figure it out. I began to argue constantly at home and imagined suicide. I transferred colleges and my grades began to drop from A's to C's.

I left my last college, becoming a cult member at a commune where my condition worsened. It was shortly after, when unable to adjust back to "reality" I suffered a first severe breakdown with deep depression. After time I recovered and returned to college.

Following this, I had a second breakdown. Living at home as a dropout, I married. During a long marriage, I worked my way through several psychotherapists including a Freudian. My constantly changing moods caused a rift and a failed business partnership. We separated, divorced, and I lost custody of my wonderful children.

After this, came fifteen years of poverty. I finally finished up college, then graduate school by working odd jobs and taking out loans. I lived on my own in a series of sad apartments with almost no friends. I was non medicated and focused on controlling myself. Most family relationships became too difficult to maintain .

In 2003, after achieving the professional certification I had long desired, I entered the work world as a teacher. My ex-spouse permitted my son to live with me. This did not last for long, as both of us shared the same predisposition. Finally, my son walked out on me.

A new breakdown occurred as I dealt with unemployment, malnutrition and some work-related injuries. I walked into a hospital while homeless suffering from depression. This led to a diagnosis of bipolar disorder I. After phasing into a Partial Program, I achieved a new found stability bolstered financially by coming into an inheritance when my last parent died.

I set myself up in an apartment and went back to work. Once again, instability led to job loss. I had applied for SSID and SSD, and knew this was my only prudent course of action as my money began to run out and my credit card debt rise.

Just when it seemed it was all over, a kind nun rescued me, gave me direction, and helped me get into debt counseling and mediation. Avoiding a third bankruptcy, (which is usually impossible), I began to learn about bipolar.

With an accurate diagnosis, with the help of a talented therapist who found me the sole effective drug to take in my case, I lifted myself up to where I am now.

I am a part time employed teacher on SSD. I have fully acknowledged my mental illness, and accept my legal disabled status. I joined NAMI, which became more relevant to my needs with every day I participated. Although I have not been able to restore family relationships in most cases, I do retain the friendship of my sister. Although there is an order of protection in effect until 2013, I do have some hope I will be able to restore a relationship with my brother and his family. My children seem a lost cause, no contact for six years and two years respectively, but I pray.

I am now a self-published author of five books, with more to come. Bipolar I seems to be in remission this Fall, and I am starting a "medication vacation" to see if I can manage on less. I have good reason to be optimistic. I have maintained my faith in God. I hope my story gives confidence and hope to others.

If you like what you read in Part 2, please visit the author's current blog at:

marykhazakgrant.wordpress.com for the latest pertinent ideas.

ABOUT THE AUTHOR:

MARY KHAZAK GRANT:

Mary Khazak Grant, B.A. Psych., M.S. Educ.-Deaf Studies

Mary Khazak Grant, age 64,   has been an artist, poet and hobby crafter from an early age.   She now works as a teacher for the Rochester Public Schools. Before coming to Rochester, New York in 2009, she spent most of her life on Long Island, New York.   Before becoming a teacher, Mary spent over twenty years in the fields of print and publishing, working as a skilled typist, typesetter, commercial paste-up artist, assistant art director and production person.   As an independent entrepreneur, she owned and managed   "Satellite Text Design", a desktop publishing business for over 12 years.   After returning to college in middle age, she completed several degrees, and became a special educator of children. These include a Bachelor's Degree in Psychology from S.U.N.Y. at Stony Brook in 1998, and a Masters of Science degree in Communication Disorders awarded in 2003 from Adelphi University, where she graduated summa cum laude.   She is a member of the Honorary Education Society Kappa Delta Pi as well as a permanently certified teacher of the deaf from the Council for Education of the Deaf. Her professional career is coupled with hobbies in textile handicrafts, stained glass design, and painting. At the present time, the author is pursuing a writing career while living up in the beautiful Finger Lakes region of Western New York State.   Check out other fine books self-published by this author at her storefront: lulu.com/spotlight/maryriver8.

NOTES:

www.ingramcontent.com/pod-product-compliance
Lightning Source LLC
Chambersburg PA
CBHW080418290526
45791CB00008BA/2326